Inspiring stories of overcor
challenges to live a fulfilling and bountiful life

Live Your
ABUNDANT
LIFE Too

Aya Fubara Eneli, Esq.

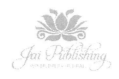

Scripture quotations taken from the Holy Bible: New International Version and King James Version Bible, unless otherwise noted. Used by permission.

Scripture quotations taken from the New American Standard Bible® (NASB), Copyright © 1960, 1962, 1963, 1968, 1971, 1972, 1973, 1975, 1977, 1995 by The Lockman Foundation. Used by permission. www.Lockman.org.

Scripture quotations taken from the Amplified® Bible (AMP), Copyright © 2015 by The Lockman Foundation. Used by permission. www.Lockman.org.

Scripture taken from the New King James Version®. Copyright © 1982 by Thomas Nelson. Used by permission. All rights reserved.

Printed in the United States of America

ISBN-13: 978-0-578-43356-1
ISBN-10: 0-578-43356-7

Contents

Introduction

by Aya Fubara Eneli, Esq.
Pioneer Author

This book is not for the faint of heart nor for those women who, for whatever reasons, are choosing to shrink into the small spaces the world demands of them.

This book is for women who have loved and lost; women who have been knocked down but have chosen to get back up again. It is a book for the brave souls who would choose to be defined not by their experiences or circumstances, but by the dreams in their hearts, the love in their souls, the wisdom in their beings, the calling of their purpose.

This is a book for anyone who has the temerity and audacity to face their fears, embrace their limitations, cloak themselves in faith, trust their instincts, obey the truth on the inside of them, and courageously reclaim and speak their power regardless of how it is received.

In a world that still chooses to subjugate and silent women, violate and defile them, beat them down, choke the life out of them, exploit them, marginalize them and spill their blood on their sheets and in the streets, these eight remarkable women have joined with me to proclaim our power. This is our declaration of independence, proof of our liberation and our herald to other women to rise and live their abundant life too.

The stories that unfold in the pages of this book cover some of the most hurtful topics and challenges that women experience. From neglect to child sexual abuse, to rape, to the stigma of poverty to divorce, the challenges of blended families, struggles with self-worth, incest, infertility, domestic violence to abortion, spousal abuse to grief – no issue is taboo, nor off limits.

In a world where women often feel compelled to suffer in silence, to be more concerned about saving the reputations of others, to allow themselves to be defined and crushed by the egos and sensitivities of those who oppress them, the eight remarkable women with whom I have collaborated on this book, have courageously chosen to share their truths. They have chosen to shed light on the secrets too many women harbor. They are lending their voices to a rising chorus of women who are saying, "We choose not just to live, we choose to thrive. We choose to live our abundant lives."

This book features the voices of a diverse group of women including veterans, educators, a physician, a social worker, a nurse, attorneys, mothers, divorcees, wives and business owners.

There are four main reasons we have chosen to share our stories, our struggles, lessons and triumphs with you. The first reason is to celebrate finding our voices and to encourage other women to reclaim their voices too. Pulitzer Prize Winner, Alice Walker, stated it best when she said, "No person is your friend who demands your silence or denies your right to grow."

You may come from one of those families where you were never supposed to share the family's secrets or "dirty laundry," but rather you were to suffer in silence, endure predators and watch the same patterns play out generation after generation in your family. You may have been convinced that you are the crazy one for believing that you have worth, that you have value and you deserve joy, love and peace. It is our hope that in the pages of this book, you will find the encouragement to speak your truth regardless of whether anyone is listening.

Our second reason for writing this book is to inspire more women to defy the power of evil to limit us by shedding a bright and public life on issues we have been taught to endure alone and in silence. We want to get rid of the shame and the stigma of our experiences. We want other women to know they are not alone, their experiences are not unique, and even though they've been knocked down, they can rise stronger and more fulfilled.

We wanted to share our fight and our journey into becoming our own best advocates. Maya Angelou reminded us of the duty we have to ourselves when she wrote, "I not only have the right to stand up for myself, but I have the responsibility. I can't ask somebody else to stand up for me if I won't stand up for myself. And once you stand up for yourself, you'd be surprised that people say, "Can I be of help?"

Our third reason for writing this book is to facilitate the healing of others. It is our prayer that millions of women will read the stories of these courageous women and they will choose to do the work to ensure their own growth and healing. Too many spend their lifetime looking for answers, healing and validation from without, but I have come to know this truth for myself, all I need is within me. I need only look within.

You must embrace your healing or your dis-ease will block the flow of your life. Your healing is the key to living a life of peace, purpose, joy and fulfillment. Your healing will determine the quality of your life and the legacy you leave. Your healing will dictate the issues that bleed into the lives of your offspring and everything else you birth. Your healing is predicated on self-love and you and you alone can determine if, when and how you choose to heal.

Finally, we have written this book to create a platform for the brilliant women who have contributed their stories to be heard around the world and to create an opportunity for each of us to do what we love on a larger stage. If you are enlightened, inspired or encouraged by their stories, share the word, promote this book and invite them to come and speak at your events.

Proceeds of this book will also help fund the Kenechukwu and Aya Eneli Foundation, and particularly the Intelligent & Talented Girls Empowerment group which is the main initiative of the Foundation.

Of the millions of books in the world, you chose this one. Honor that choice. Find and celebrate your voice. Embrace your story. Pursue your healing. Choose to **Live Your Abundant Life Too!**

🦋 🦋 🦋 🦋

Chapter One

When Life Makes No Sense

by Aya Fubara Eneli, Esq.

> *Your history is not just a tale of the past, it should also serve as a frame of reference to chart a more excellent future.*
>
> *Aya Fubara Eneli*

I threw the journal across the room trying to get it as far away from me as possible. I couldn't talk, not that there was anyone there to talk to. I was all alone in the house. Everyone else was living their normal lives, going to work, taking classes, caring for kids. But my life, on the good days, felt like it was at a literal standstill. On the bad days, it was like I had fallen into quicksand, the more I struggled to hold on to my sanity, the deeper I sunk.

In the silence of the house, every sound was magnified. I could hear the refrigerator humming in the kitchen, the leaves rustling in the tree right outside my window, the gentle movements of our aging family home. I buried my head in the pillows and pulled the comforter over my head in an attempt to drown out the sounds. All I succeeded in doing so was creating an echo chamber for the loudest sound of all—the thump, thump, thump of my heart. Louder and louder it got like the drums of my ancestral home.

What should have flooded me with memories of happier times, instead filled me with dread. I prayed. I cried. I tried to sleep. I hoped it was just a nightmare from which I would awaken. But it was broad daylight and I was wide awake, and this "mare" needed neither night nor sleep to terrorize me. It had bullied and intimidated me for the better of two years. It had taken great pleasure at pulverizing my hopes and dreams, stripping me of my confidence, robbing me of my joy, mocking my plans, playing with my mind, stomping on my emotions, stomping like it wanted to take me out for good.

I stayed in bed all day willing myself to stay still, legs propped up while I prayed. I got up only to use the bathroom and each time I wiped, I would look down with relief at the clear tissue. I heard cars drive up and doors open. My three-year old son ran into the room and immediately jumped in the bed to hug and kiss me.

"Are you feeling better, mommy?" He asked. How should I answer him? Do I smile and reassure him, or do I tell him the truth that was filling me with such dread?

The next morning, I woke up and headed to the bathroom. Today was a bad day. I was sinking and sinking fast. My heart had not stopped thumping and I instinctively knew what was coming next. I made my way carefully to the bathroom all the while hoping and praying against hope. As I pulled down my underwear, my heart caught in my throat. I let out a scream only I could hear as I looked down at the blood that seemed to be everywhere. My cousin must have heard some sound because she came rushing into the unlocked bathroom. She saw, screamed and ran to get my mother.

I don't remember how I got dressed or made my way to the car, but somehow, we were racing to the hospital, my mother behind the wheel all but running red lights. I could see myself rocking back and forth in the back seat of my mother's Mazda. I was humming Christian choruses from my childhood underneath my breath. My cousin, Isobel, was praying out loud and trying to reassure me. My mother was freaking out. We made it to the hospital and I was wheeled into an exam room and placed on the table. I was calm as scalding tears ran down my cheeks and pooled around my ears. I was still humming. I already knew the outcome. My baby was dead. The only question was, "Why was I still alive?"

I held my lifeless 14-week old baby in my hand. He was a boy. You could tell from his penis. He also had all ten fingers and toes. I named him Chukwuemeka –

God has done exceedingly well. The tears came faster and hotter. I kept expecting to take my last breath and join my four children now in Heaven, but death laughed and left the room. I relived the events of the last 24 hours.

>‖> >‖> >‖>

My journal had been my constant companion through my time on bedrest. I had gotten sick almost as soon as I got pregnant. My physicians took all precautions putting me on bedrest, progesterone and other vitamins and steroids designed to ensure I carried this baby to term and had a healthy child. After having our son, we had endured three miscarriages (I hate that word) in a row. Being on bedrest was torture for an active person and I struggled to quiet my mind. I read and wrote incessantly.

The day before, I was in a particularly melancholy mood when I wrote these words, "Lord, if I lose this baby I know I will just die. I can't take any more pain." The minute I wrote those words, a sense of dread came over me. I literally felt like I had just opened the door to evil and had exposed my greatest vulnerability. I heard a voice say, "Curse God and you and your baby will live." I was reminded of Job's wife who advised him to just curse God. It was then that I threw my journal. But it was too late, the damage had already been done.

After my D&C (Dilation and Curettage) procedure, my mother and cousin left so I could get some rest. I had to stay overnight in the hospital. My husband who had been away at a conference in Canada, cut his trip short and was struggling to make his way back to me. I was alone again with nothing but my torturous thoughts when the phone rang. It was my older brother. We must have exchanged pleasantries, but I have no recollection of that. All I remember as sure as it was yesterday were these words, "When are you going to get righteously angry?" I am not sure if I hung up the phone on him, but I was so livid I was shaking. How dare he? How dare he imply that I was somehow responsible for losing my babies? What mother purposely chooses to get pregnant and then lose four children?

His words seared my heart and I was angry. Angry at him. Angry at God. Angry at my body for betraying me yet again. Angry at my cousins who had sexually molested me as a child. Angry at the world. It was so unfair. And to top it all, God wouldn't just take me as well. Here I was, left behind, to feel it all...the nonstop unbearable pain of so much loss in such a short period of time. I was devastated. I was so distressed that I couldn't focus or function at work. I was so shattered that on more than one occasion I woke up only to realize I had urinated on myself.

Since I hadn't died from the grief and pain like I had anticipated, I had to figure out what to do with my life, if not for myself, then for the sake of my young son. This began my search for meaning. Out of the depths of my despair I challenged God to give me beauty for my ashes, joy for my mourning and to return to me what the locusts had devoured so I could experience the abundant life. It was out of my incredible loss that my first book, Live Your Abundant Life, was birthed and fourteen years later, I am hoping this book encourages you no matter your circumstances. There are many lessons I have gleaned from this tragic period in my life. I share these lessons with you to encourage, empower and equip you to rise above your "mares" and live your abundant life too.

>⫸ >⫸ >⫸

Honestly, it is really hard to write this. I don't want to relive the pain of those years. I don't want to remember a despair so deep that I contemplated ending my life. I don't want to replay the sleepless nights on a drenched pillow. I don't want to go back to the overwhelming sense of loss I felt as the miscarriages piled up. I wanted to hold it all together. I was told that since they hadn't lived outside of the womb, I really hadn't lost any children. Others assured me that God was trying to protect me because my babies would most likely have been developmentally impaired. I had a son depending on me. I had a job with deadlines and responsibilities. Besides, strong women don't fall apart. Christians don't despair. Black women don't have the luxury of mental breakdowns. I was 29 years old, a professional, an African woman with great promise, I couldn't afford to fall apart. I put up a brave front, though I was falling apart. Fortunately, I did not stay that way; my healing began one day in a thunderstorm.

Own Your Truth

My neighbor had kindly taken my toddler son to an evening kids' program at their church. My husband was at the hospital on a residency rotation and would be there all night. I was home alone. The sky was overcast and dark gray. It suited my state of mind perfectly. I had just had what would be the first of many D&C procedures and I was completely out of sorts.

I stared out the window of my beautiful middle-class home as the rain drops started falling, slow and intermittently and then faster and faster. I watched my tears drop and begin to pool on my kitchen counter. I named each tear. This one was for my baby, gone too soon. This one was for my hopes and dreams for the child I would not see on this earth. This one was for my well-meaning colleague who said I was still young and could have more. This one was for the paralyzing sense of hopelessness that had wrapped itself around me like a too snug sweater dress. This one was because it wasn't supposed to happen to me. This one was for my anger towards God. This one …this one was for the fear that my sins had caught up with me.

And on that revelation, my internal dam broke just as a thunderous light split the darkened sky. My tears became a raging torrent pounding my head, scalding my senses, ripping me apart and in desperation I ran out in the rain daring the lightening to end it all. I screamed at God and I returned thunder with thunder. I unleashed my anger, my fear and the unfairness of it all.

I don't know how long I was out there. I don't know if my neighbors saw me. I really didn't care if they had. After a while, I made my way back into my home, the storm within and without had abated. All that was left was the truth of my circumstances, like the water clinging to my hair, running down my back and pooling around my feet.

I was devastated. It was okay to be devastated. It was okay not to be fully functional. It was okay to take time to grieve. It was okay to lose it without warning like when I saw a pregnant woman or heard a baby's cry or got an invitation to a Baby Shower in the mail. It was okay not to have an appetite in one moment and in another to eat a whole apple pie with vanilla ice cream. My truth was that I was not coping so well, and I was no longer going to try to wear a mask to make others feel more comfortable.

I wasn't going to keep my loss a secret either. When I had my first miscarriage, I was surprised to find out that one out of four pregnancies ends in a miscarriage. That statistic was a surprise to me. No one around me had ever talked about losing a child in vitro or infertility. My mother had seven children. It never occurred to me that I wouldn't and couldn't carry a healthy baby to term.

Nonetheless, here I was. I decided not to hide my grief. Many times, I stayed away from people rather than put on a façade. At other times, I gave voice to my pain. Owning the truth of my brokenness and despair was the first step to my healing. Giving myself permission to grieve my loss accelerated my healing. What truth about yourself or your circumstances are you denying?

Harvesting the Value in the Valley

There is a Bible verse that really challenged me as I sought to make sense of my losses. Romans 8:28 (King James Version) states, "And we know that all things work together for good to those who love God, to those who are called according to His purpose." As I endured not one, not two, not three, but FOUR consecutive miscarriages, I struggled to make sense of where God was and what lesson(s), if any, I was to glean from my great misfortune. What possible good could come out of all these tragedies, all this pain? How could any good come out of such immense and irrevocable loss?

Looking back now, I can honestly say that a tremendous amount of good has grown out of the losses I suffered. While I wouldn't wish what I experienced on my worst enemy, I am the woman and mother I am today because of the insights I gained from my extended time in the valley. The valley was my place of deep despair where I hardly allowed anyone to penetrate. It's where I cried and thought about my life and future.

My losses caused me to examine every aspect of my life. I began to question my choices and my understanding of myself. I examined everything I could think of – my faith, my marriage, my childhood, my education choices, my career, my friendships, my beliefs and philosophy about life, my future goals, hopes and dreams. This introspection served me well as I discovered depths to myself I had previously overlooked. I also realized that I had past traumas that I had buried and from which I had never healed. I decided to live my life intentionally as opposed to just doing what society expected of me regardless of whether it lined up with my vision for my life. Years later, I would get certified as a Life Coach and create a survey for others to take inventory of their lives, so they could live intentionally.

In my valley, I found clarity. Clarity of purpose, clarity for how to live the rest of my life. I realized I wasn't just on earth to work and pay bills and occasionally have some fun. I had a specific assignment to inspire and empower and equip girls and women live to their highest potential. I knew to achieve that aim I must first empower myself to be my best. I have been on that quest ever since and can say that as I grow, I have facilitated the healing and growth of many others.

One major impact of my time in the valley has been to recognize the fragility of life and how fortunate we are for any opportunities to love. Since my miscarriages, we have been blessed with four more living children, making me a mother of five. Although it takes a lot of hard work and sacrifice to raise five children, I am grateful for every moment I get to be a mother to my children. I am intentional about everything I do with them and by God's grace they've all thrived and are really great kids.

My career and ambitions have taken a backseat to parenting in this season of my life, but I am unperturbed. I know I am doing exactly what I should be doing as I wholeheartedly embrace the fleeting opportunity to shape their lives. I am a better mother, a more loving wife, and I enjoy a stronger relationship with my Creator as a result of the clarity I received in my time in the valley.

The value I found in my valley also led to a change in careers for me. Although trained as an attorney, I have always been drawn to helping women be their best selves. I taught time and stress management workshops in college and facilitated seminars for women. After my last miscarriage, I quit my job and after some soul-searching began writing a weekly column in my local newspaper titled 'Live Your Abundant Life'. That column led to a best-selling book by the same title and increased speaking and training opportunities for me. I have been self-employed ever since. Today, I get to coach and empower women all over the world and help them overcome their challenges, find the value in their valley and live their abundant lives.

Tapping the Power Within

How do you value you? How do you see you? What do you see as possible for yourself? When you think of your future are they optimistic thoughts or are they fraught with the fear of your experiences? Are your choices powered by all that is possible or hindered by all that could go wrong? Do you tend to focus on what you currently lack, or on who you could grow into that would eliminate that lack? James Allen famously said, "As a man thinketh, so is he."

My miscarriages literally and figuratively brought me to my knees. I wanted to die. Nothing made sense in my life anymore. I felt powerless and out of control. I wanted to end it all and have some peace. I also knew that was a selfish thought. But, my pain was so great, and I just wanted to feel better. I just wanted to feel normal again.

One Fall morning, as I sat in our new and unfurnished home in Illinois, I had what experts will call both a breakdown and a breakthrough. I was in particularly bad shape that day. The tears wouldn't stop falling, I was hurt and angry and I wanted someone or something to blame.

Suddenly, I felt like there was a presence in the room with me. It was a soothing voice telling me that I needed to break free of my depression and choose to really live again. Yelling in the empty room, I recounted every harrowing experience, the joy of discovering I was pregnant, the horror of seeing the blood and knowing the worst had happened, the ultrasounds with technicians who leave the room with promises of bringing a doctor to tell me my results, the anguish of telling yet another person that I was no longer pregnant.

The voice heard me out and then told me I had a choice. "You are standing at a crossroads. You can choose the path of anger and despair, shame and guilt or you can choose the path of joy and an abundant life."

As the voice spoke, I was reminded of an older relative of mine who had lost her husband in her youth. In all the years I had known her, I never saw her smile or laugh genuinely. She and her pain had become one. There was no joy in her. She was surrounded by people who loved her, but I never saw her let anyone in. I knew then, I didn't want her life. But what did an abundant life mean and how was I supposed to get there from here?

When I think of an abundant life, I think of a life of purpose, joy, love, intentionality. I think of health and not just the absence of lack, but an overflow of everything I need to thrive and give to others. An abundant life is not free of challenges, but it is a mindset that allows one to always focus on how to overcome and utilize one's adversities. An abundant life flows out of the quality of one's thoughts for as a woman thinketh, so is she. Her thoughts feed her emotions. Her emotions guide her actions. Her actions determine her results.

While I have known of this quote for a significant amount of time, in these days as I get older, it has taken on much more significance to me. As I take inventory of my life, everything, and I mean everything I am, have or experienced is directly linked to my thoughts. In other words, if there are areas in my life that bring me great pleasure, they are because of my thoughts. Likewise, if there is any lack, pain, dysfunction in my life, that too is directly tied to my thoughts as well.

So, rather than believing I have just been lucky or cursing at my misfortunes, the more helpful question is, "What have I been thinking and how do I ensure that my thoughts are in line with what I claim I want to see in my life?"

Here is a radical thought from Author, Life Coach and TV personality, Iyanla Vanzant, " We cannot outperform our level of self-esteem. We cannot draw to ourselves more than we think we are worth."

My miscarriages were not my fault, but how I choose to think about and react to the events of my life is totally within my power, if I choose to exercise it. Take a moment to examine yourself in light of this statement. Haven't you always made choices based on what you believe is possible for you? How often have you said, "I can't do that!" Or, "I am no good at ...." What happened when you thought and said that? Can you see how you live up to your thoughts?

A few years ago, during one of our family discussions on John Maxwell's book, Intentional Living, I posed a question to my 8-year-old son as we grappled with the consequences of some poor choices he had been making recently. He had traced his actions back to what he was thinking at the time and so I asked, "Where do your thoughts come from?" We explored a variety of answers and finally we agreed that there is a lot of information always floating around us and our thoughts are those ideas, words and information that we choose to pull out from everything around us and focus on.

We likened it to having a TV capable of accessing hundreds of channels, but we don't have to watch every channel, rather, the person with the remote has the power to decide what channel to watch and for how long. That person can reject a channel whenever they so choose. The same is true for you and me. We have the power to choose what ideas we focus on and plant in our minds. We have the power to choose what to believe. Whatever we choose to focus on becomes a force that either attracts or repels people, things and experiences.

Medical practitioners will tell you about the power of "the will to live". Patients who have the will to live because of the quality of their thoughts, always have better chances of recovery than patients with a negative mindset. The thoughts of a person can actually determine whether they live or die. How powerful is that?

James Allen says, "Man is made or unmade by himself. All that a man (and a woman) achieves and all that he fails to achieve is the direct result of his own thoughts." Wow! Again, I ask. How do you value you? How do you see you? What do you see as possible for yourself? When you think of your future are they optimistic thoughts or are they fraught with the fear of your perceived limitations?

I realize now that I create my life with my thoughts. My life is impacted by the circumstances of my birth, my education, my gender, hue and ethnicity and by things beyond my control like losing my babies. But, more than anything, my thoughts have created my life and how I feel about my life. If I want better, I must tap the power within me to think better thoughts. As I think, so shall I be. As you think, so shall you be. Tap into the power to choose your thoughts.

The Company You Keep

Have you ever read the story about Job in the Bible? He was suddenly beset by troubles on all sides.

He lost everything – his wealth, status and children. He had some friends around him who were not at all helpful. In fact, if he had followed their advice, things would have worked out even worse for him.

In the depths of my despair, I started paying close attention to the people around me and how they made me feel. I tell you no lie when I say some of them seemed to revel in my misery. Some were dismissive of my pain. Some loved me to the point that their love weakened versus strengthening me. Others seized the opportunity to point out all the ways in which they thought I had brought on my own losses.

One pastor told me it was a sign from God to not be career-oriented. Another pastor tried to convince me that my enemies had unleashed evil against me and were eating my babies in my womb! I declined when he tried to lay hands on me to pray the evil out.

But, I was also fortunate to have some amazing people in my life who constantly reminded me that I am much more than my circumstances. They encouraged me to figure out how to use my pain and experiences to do more good in the world. "You are still alive, aren't you?" One would ask. "Well, live like it!"

Show me your friends and I will tell you who you are. The company we keep absolutely impacts how we see the world and what choices we make. If you want to live an abundant life you must determine to keep company with only those who have already accomplished what you are seeking, or those who are diligently pursuing similar goals. Too often we get into a comfort zone by seeking out happy-go-lucky people who have no goals and ambitions, and those whom we know look up to us. Or worse, we settle with those who think lowly of us and tell us we will amount to nothing.

When you hit hardships, it is more important than ever to carefully choose your company. Think about it this way: Imagine you have just had major surgery and your immune system had been compromised, that is no time to invite any and everybody to come and visit you. Why? Because you are more susceptible to diseases and even a common cold germ could be what causes your death.   That is the time to take precautions, to limit your exposure and give yourself time to heal. That is the time to be intentional about who you allow in your space.

Every athlete knows that they must take on the best to become good enough to one day be the best. The same applies to those who want to live an abundant life. By all means, love everyone. Don't snob people because their aspirations differ from yours. However, you must also find that core group of individuals who inspire and motivate and encourage and challenge you to become a better version of yourself.

One of the most important decisions you can make to improve your chance for a life of joy, health and success is to carefully choose the company you keep. As Tony Robbins put it, "You become the average of the five people you spend the most time with."

Look around you. Who do you call for advice? Who is your BFF? Who are your co-workers? Who are your lunch buddies? Who is your party crew or road dog? With whom do you worship? Who do you call when you need to laugh or cry? Who do you date? Who shares your bed?

The fable is told about an eagle who thought he was a chicken. When the eagle was very young, it fell from the safety of its nest. A chicken farmer found the eagle, brought it to the farm, and raised it in a chicken coop among his many chickens. The eagle grew up doing what chickens do, living like a chicken, and believing it was a chicken.

A naturalist came to the chicken farm to see if what he had heard about an eagle acting like a chicken was true. He knew that an eagle is king of the sky. He was surprised to see the eagle strutting around the chicken coop, pecking at the ground, and acting very much like a chicken. The farmer explained to the naturalist that this bird was no longer an eagle. It was now a chicken because it had been trained to be a chicken and the eagle believed that it was a chicken.

The naturalist was distraught and wanted the eagle to realize the great potential in itself and so he asked the farmer's permission to work with the eagle. The farmer was convinced the eagle will always think and act like a chicken. The first two times the naturalist attempted to set the eagle free, it just ignored the man and went back to pecking like the other chicken.

The naturalist tried a third time and this time, he took the eagle away from the chicken coop and the farmhouse and all it was comfortable with. The man held the eagle on his arm and pointed high into the sky where the bright sun was beckoning above. He spoke: "Eagle, thou art an eagle! Thou dost belong to the sky and not to the earth. Stretch forth thy wings and fly." This time the eagle stared skyward into the bright sun, straightened its large body, and stretched its massive wings. Its wings moved, slowly at first, then surely and powerfully. With the mighty screech of an eagle, it flew.

While just a fable, wise people have long known this secret that the company you keep will always rub off on and impact your thoughts and therefore your actions. With this awareness, I am constantly monitoring what and to whom I am exposed because I understand the power of influence. My grandfather used to say, "Show me your friends and I'll tell you who you will be." The Bible says in 1 Corinthians 15:33 that "Bad company corrupts."

"Surround yourself with the dreamers and the doers, the believers and thinkers, but most of all, surround yourself with those who see greatness within you, even when you don't see it yourself." The Book of Proverbs 13:20 states, "He who walks with wise men will be wise, but the companion of fools will suffer harm."

The power of the company we keep is well-documented and has even resulted in business people specifically planning Mastermind Groups to not only influence their success, but also to enhance their collective capacity to excel. The choices we make regarding the company we keep speaks volumes about our values, both positively and negatively. Hang around with people with compromised values and small dreams and you will inevitably begin to take on their values and thoughts and reap similar results in your life.

When a person hangs around with other enterprising people, they become more enterprising. When a person keeps company with the wealthy, they pick up tips to begin building their own wealth. When a rich person embraces the company of the lazy and poverty-minded, he or she will eventually lose their fortune. When a person hangs around people who want them to remain victims of their circumstances, they remain victims instead of becoming overcomers. In all times, but specifically in your dark hours, mind the company you keep.

Practice Gratitude

Four dead babies. Four dead babies and you are asking me to be grateful? Grateful for what? I don't know about your situation, but amid my tragedies, gratitude was the last thing on my mind. I was much more acquainted with anger, resentment, fear, despair and resignation.

I had long read about the importance of gratitude. I believed that gratitude was the key to a joyful heart.

I believed that we reaped what we sowed and if I sowed gratitude, I would reap more things for which I could be grateful. The Bible taught me to give thanks in all things. But, I sure struggled with this one this time. With each loss, it got harder and harder and harder to be grateful. I was so consumed by all I had lost, I couldn't see anything else.

The teenaged girl sulked as she trailed her mother. Every once in a while, she would speed up just to barrage her mom with a series of whys. Why can't I ever get what I want? Why do you have to be mean all the time? Why was I born into this family? Why don't you want me to be happy?

I watched the scene as it unfolded trying to piece together the reason for this young lady's apparent distress. She looked to be about 16 years old. She was fashionably dressed in the current trends of the day. Her face seemed expertly made up and in her hand was a smartphone that she would furiously type on in between her tirades. She looked well-fed and taken care of, but we all know looks don't tell the whole story.

As they made their way closer to me, I got more of the gist of the story. Her parents were getting her a car for the holidays, but it wasn't the car she had set her heart on. She was determined to get what she wanted.

Her frazzled mother just kept repeating, "You should really work on being more thankful."

My thoughts returned to me. Sure, I had experienced great losses, but was I overlooking my blessings in the process? Could I come up with 100 reasons to be grateful despite my losses? I decided to try. It was slow going at first. I wrote down things like, my husband, my son, my family, food, clothes, a roof over my head, my education, my job, my eyes, my hands .... you get the idea. I imagined my life without my health and all the opportunities I had. I realized that like that teenage girl, I was being quite ungrateful. Even in my current circumstances, what would life look, feel, sound, and even smell like if I committed to not just occasionally being thankful, but actually living in a perpetual state of gratitude, of thankfulness. But, what does that mean?

Webster's dictionary defines thankful as, "being or showing gratitude." From that, one can deduce that we become grateful or show gratitude to the extent that we are receiving something. However, I find the synonyms of thankful even more enlightening: joyful, blissful, delighted, gratified, happy, joyous, pleased, satisfied, glad. These are emotions and ways of being that do not have to be tied to being the recipient of anything in particular. It is just a state of being.

The antonyms of thankful are also insightful: displeased, dissatisfied, joyless, sad, unhappy, unpleased, unsatisfied. Which words best capture how you live your life day in and day out?

I realized that I could choose how to live despite my experiences. I was tired of feeling bad. I believe that living in a state of thankfulness is a decision made independently of our situations. The Bible says in 1 Thessalonians 5:18 (New International Version), "Give thanks in all circumstances; for this is God's will for you in Christ Jesus." That means that we remain thankful no matter our circumstances. We are thankful when there is plenty and thankful in scarcity. We are thankful in health and thankful in sickness or death. Our state always remains the same.

I am reminded of the world-renown ice skater, Scott Hamilton, who, at the time of this writing, has battled brain cancer, not once, not twice, but three times! He admitted that he could rail against the unfairness of it all, but he had chosen a different path. Hamilton chose to celebrate and be thankful for life. He shared, "I teach students in my skating academy to get back up again and to choose to live and skate with joy." Despite his challenges, Hamilton stays thankful for what has been and what is and is hopeful for what will be.

I decided then that I would live with gratitude. I would find the joy in my daily existence and I would magnify that joy for me and those around me. I will be grateful for my life by being the best me I know to be and inspiring others to do the same. How is it that I miscarried four babies and then birthed four perfect, healthy and amazing children? I believe a grateful heart turned my life around. What do you believe? What will you do?

Into every life some rain will fall. It is not a matter of IF misfortune or challenges will befall you, it is a matter of WHEN. The question you must ask and answer for yourself is how you will choose to show up in your life when adversity strikes. I hope you will choose to own your truth, find the value in your valley, tap the immense power that lies within you, even as you exercise wisdom in the company you keep and that finally, you choose to live a life of gratitude. Whatever your circumstances, it is my hope that you choose to live your abundant life too.

Chapter Two

Abundant Change

by Keiko Anderson, Esq.

I can do all things through Christ which strengtheneth me.

Philippians 4:13 (KJV)

I am no psychic, but I guarantee you can relate to at least one of the next few statements: You have been hurt. You've been disappointed. You have had failures, and even in your victories, you have had struggles along the way. In some capacity or another you have been mistreated, rejected, used, and/or abused—if your life has been anything like mine.

I know this kind of "life" all too well. In fact, I have experienced every single one of these pains even by the age of three years old. I will tell you more about that later. I know that some of what you have faced and even what you are going through now leads you to believe that living an abundant life is a dream or a fairytale. At this point you may see so many obstacles that your faith in a bright future is failing, but I assure you there is a way to create a winning and abundant life even in the face of bad facts. Practicing family law for fifteen years has taught me this truth.

I figured out that even in a winning case, there are bad facts. Many days my office consisted of me behind my desk taking notes diligently on my yellow pad as I listened to the trembling voice of a distraught parent or spouse go through the details of every flaw and weakness in their case. In the conversation, there were moments when I casually looked across my desk only to see the person sitting across from me staring outside the office windows with the stain of defeat in their eyes.

You may not be a lawyer but if you are anyone's friend, you may have been on either side of similar conversations and you realized this—recounting the negative aspects of life inevitably brings even the strongest people to a place of defeat. We have a natural tendency to allow the low points of our lives to overtake our spirit. Some of us are convinced in these times that perhaps we are destined for a defeated life. These are the times that we have to remind ourselves that although we have obvious challenges, we can still be successful. There are strengths that we have yet to identify, strategies we have yet to form, choices we have yet to make, and changes we have yet to implement that will bring us to our desired end.

The key to securing your abundant life rests inside of you. You possess the power within to create an environment where an abundant life can flourish, but you must be intentional about creating it and willing to change current behaviors that hinder abundant living. Exercising your power to change just a few things about the way you think, feel, and behave will set the stage for your abundant life to manifest itself. Not only are you going to have to change, but it is helpful if you make some changes quickly because life is short and it gets shorter every second of the day.

⋙ ⋙ ⋙

Sometimes it hits me like a splash of cold water across your face in the early morning, just how limited time is. My godson taught me this truth. We call him Z, which is short for Zealand. Z had a smile that lit any room and his love for Christ and people coupled with his athletic build, curly hair, infectious smile, and positivity made me a proud godmother.

On Friday, June 24th, I planned to make sure to drop by his place in San Antonio, Texas since I was already in town for a carnival. On my way home from the carnival, I decided I would just wait until Sunday since he and I already had a date for church scheduled. I got home early Friday evening and settled into bed and then my phone rang. It was late enough in the evening that my whole house was quiet and I felt the uneasiness we all feel when your phone rings just a little too late for comfort. I reached across my bed and answered the phone, hearing the still voice of his mother, "Zealand has been shot."

Not only had he been shot, but he had been shot multiple times. He was shot in his head, his throat and his chest multiple times at point blank range. Some part of me had faith that somehow he would survive this. He was only 20 years old and so strong. In my mind he was going to make it, and he had to. After all, we had plans. Church on Sunday. Brunch after church. But the truth was that he had no chance of survival and he died on the curb of a dark San Antonio street.

I became angry with myself. I should have stopped by to see him on my way home from the carnival. If I had, maybe he would not have gone to the place where he was murdered. I thought I had plenty of time to see Z and it would be fine to wait until our Sunday date. I thought I had two days to see him, but it turned out that I only had about six hours left to see him alive. That's how short life is.

June 24th was a day that I knew from the deepest part of my soul that I must make every effort to live every one of the days I have left to its fullest potential. Understanding this gives me every reason to be urgently motivated to move toward an abundantly filled life of love, joy, and peace. You and I must commit to pursuing the best that life has to offer and we must make changes that bring us nearer to that destination now.

>⼁⊳ >⼁⊳ >⼁⊳

Change what? You might ask. Change your mind. Change your heart. Change your actions. Then change your view, your response, and your company.

Change Your Mind

The first thing you can change is your mindset. Changing your mindset in areas that you have found to be unproductive in moving you toward your best life will be necessary in order to create an environment for an abundant life. You may need to change your mindset about priorities, money, politics, or other things. I can tell you that I had to change my mentality specifically about people.

Until recent years, I was a huge fan of isolation strategies. Since my early years, I consistently told myself things like, "I can do bad by myself" or "I'm not a people person." When I was old enough to learn about personality traits, I labeled myself an introvert to justify the truth that I was afraid of trusting people.

I decided that engaging others was a sure way to destruction.

My past was a testament to the fact that people were terrible. My father left my mother and myself when I was two years old. He abandoned me, and apart from a few choice cameo appearances (graduation and my second wedding), he was an absentee parent.

My father's father molested me in nauseating ways from the age of three to six years old. By the time I was six years old, I knew more than most adults about pornography, foreplay, digital manipulation, intercourse, sex toys, and sexual deviancy. Not only was I well versed in sexual activity, but on a nightly basis I was forced to drink excessive amounts of Cognac as I sat in my childhood pajamas at my kid-sized pink plastic kitchen table, waiting for my grandfather's next instruction. He was later arrested and sentenced to serve his time in the penitentiary, so I was freed physically from the abuse but not psychologically. I didn't trust anyone.

The instability in my home did not help matters. I was one of three children and all of us had different fathers. Another man was my first stepfather and he was an alcoholic which brought all sorts of negativity into our home—from interrupted employment to vehicular accidents to bar brawls and eventually to my mother's divorce. That left me in a single parent home with a working mother and all too many days and nights taking care of my younger brother. My younger brother then grew up to be a drug addict which left me his caretaker in many ways well into adulthood. I identified with no one in my family and I connected with no one other than my maternal grandmother, who suffered from depression and she died when I was young.

As a result of abuse and disappointment with people, I decided that my best life would be a life lived alone where I could trust that no one would hurt me. I purposed to separate myself from people. I buried myself in academia. I was quite intelligent and enjoyed the challenge of academia. I excelled naturally. My joy was found in my accomplishments in school but I shared the joy with no one.

I remember being told that my door would be removed from the hinges if I kept going in my room and closing myself away from the rest of the household. I didn't care. That would not matter to me; because I was so gifted, I learned how to isolate myself from people emotionally even if I was unable to escape them physically. It took me a long time to figure out that I was so busy not being hurt by people, that I was hurting myself.

>» >» >»

Fast forward two decades. After many failed relationships and a divorce, I met DeVry. Everything I learned about love, he taught me. My husband loved me through my dysfunctional mindset and showed me that there are people who are sent by God to enrich and add value to our lives if we open ourselves to love. This was the beginning of my journey toward an abundant life.

Sure I had accolades and degrees. I was the one in my family who had "made it", and I was the one that all of my friends came to for advice. Many people would probably consider me to have had an abundant life at that time, but I didn't. Not by my definition. I was living life with the wrong mindset, and to move toward a truly fulfilled life I had to change my mind about people. I chose to adopt a new mind that valued people and acknowledged the need for relationship with others.

>» >» >»

If you have convinced yourself that you are better living life alone with your independent self, please reconsider. There is no chance of an abundant life in isolation. There is no such thing as a person who became successful alone. It is counter to who you were naturally and spiritually created to be to walk alone.

If you become intentional about changing any part of your mindset that minimizes the value of people and relationships, then you will begin to recognize the benefits in every relationship, even the strained ones. You will find there is an opportunity for introspection and personal growth in every relationship.

As you spend more of your time addressing the weaknesses in yourself, and less time rehearsing the faults of others, then every relationship can become an instrument for your growth, which enhances the quality of your life. You will then find yourself living more abundantly.

>I> >I> >I>

Now that you know you need to enlist others into your life in order to have a beautiful life, you may have to change some of your perspectives about yourself in the context of relationships. Before I changed my perspective, I operated in most relationships from the perspective of "I am right." This is a dangerous perspective to have if you want to maintain unity with others. Looking at relationships from this perspective makes one person right and the other person wrong and creates division.

Instead, adopt the perspective of "we are different" or "we disagree." I have decided to replace "I am right" with "I am kind." One method I've implemented is taking a moment to see things from the other person's perspective. Even in the largest disagreements, if you take a moment to put yourself in the other person's position, you will often find yourself empathizing with them and understanding them better. Focusing your attention on others and how they view things helps you to reconnect and ultimately improves the quality of your life. It minimizes the number of broken relationships you will have.

Look at your life. Are you disconnected from people that you used to enjoy because of insignificant disagreements? Remember that people are different. People think and feel differently than you. This is a positive thing. An abundant life is a life of loving people who are different than you, as well as those who are similar to you. This practice can help bridge the gap between you and others and it has improved the quality of my life drastically.

Change Your Heart

Your heart is another critical area to examine and change. There is no chance of a fulfilled life with a hardened heart. I found out that abundant life is not found in material wealth alone. An abundant life will require your heart to be free from unforgiveness and bitterness. A heart open to love and filled with compassion brings out the richest parts of life.

I spent many months living a materialistically abundant life, yet an emotionally drained life due to a bitter heart. There were more nights than I can count falling asleep next to a doting husband, in a luxury home with every amenity, multiple cars, money in various bank accounts, flourishing businesses, beautiful friends, and the greatest church family, yet was unfulfilled because I let one family member offend me to the point of lingering resentment for months.

I am naturally a giver. I am naturally a caretaker. I do it without thinking but when I found myself giving to someone who I felt had no appreciation, I found myself struggling to forgive and, as a result, I found myself living a life of bitterness—until I changed my heart.

⇶ ⇶ ⇶

It started off so beautifully. This bitterness crept its way inside my heart in the context of blending families. Of course I walked into my second marriage completely blind to the possibility that a child would not accept me. I was the child whisperer. There was not a child I met that I didn't like or didn't like me. It just wasn't one of my problems. I work with children. I've been in children's ministry for years.

Then at the altar in my beautiful wedding dress standing with the man of my dreams, the pastor called our children up to light unity candles with us. We all approached the unity candle with our individual lighters and one child began uncontrollably sobbing with tears. I realized then that I had missed something. These were not happy tears. These were devastated tears. I could see it. From that day forward, I spent the first few years of my marriage playing the role of a mother to a child who was bent on rejecting me in that position.

Unfortunately, I was the only option because the biological mother was completely absent. The longer we did life together as a family, the more I resented the fact that I was working and providing every physical necessity for a child who showed no appreciation or gratitude. I was beyond angry. I didn't show it because that would not be ladylike, but I was silently livid.

How could you reject me and you have no other option? Don't you know how much worse your life would be without me? Every arrogant spirit rested in my heart after every meal I made, every ride to school, every errand shopping for clothes, every doctor appointment. Every motherly duty I performed with resentment in my heart, and it stole the joy of the blessed life I had.

I had to change my heart. I had to create a space in my heart for compassion for a child who lost their mother suddenly and entirely. I had to remember that I was a child born into a broken home with no father and the lack I experienced. I had to remember the loneliness there is when you feel like the disconnected child in a home.

That was me. I was raised in a home with no father, and then an alcoholic father, and then a father I did not accept. As I reconsidered the issues I was having in a blended family as a stepmother, I tapped into the compassionate part of my heart and remembered myself as the stepchild in order to try to be more understanding. I suddenly found so many likenesses that it was shocking. I immediately went to my family and expressed my desire to improve our relationship and move forward in love.

If you saw us today, you would think we had intense counseling and therapy. We moved from just tolerating each other to genuine love and concern for each other. We laugh and talk and enjoy each other. We have an abundant life now, and it grew from a place of various forms of death. Death of a prior marriage, death of a dream of being parented by natural parents, death of a stepmother's expectation of a perfect blended family, and more importantly death of harboring resentment and bitterness in my heart toward a hurting child made room for an abundant life to flourish.

Changing your heart about the very thing that is stealing your joy in this moment and deciding to find a way to accept and understand the things that hurt you the most will actually set you free. An abundant life is a life that is lived in freedom.

Change Your Actions

Next, change your actions. Changing your actions has to be in combination with changing your heart and changing your mind. You must change your mind and your heart first, otherwise your actions will be fraudulent and meaningless, and will not bring you to your desired end of living an abundant life.

Change Your View

I suggest that the first action you take after changing your mind and heart is to change the way you view problems. Remember that you may have problems but they do not have you unless you give them authority. Convince yourself that you are able to recover and overcome every problem either alone or by enlisting the help of others.

The process of overcoming trials begins with a decision within yourself to attack the issue and an expectation within yourself that you will succeed. I have decided that in every circumstance, I will not be defeated or discouraged. I see myself in the future telling the story to others of how I conquered whatever issue. This gives me motivation to fight harder and not to give up.

If you take a moment to zoom out of the smallness of an individual trial, you begin to see the larger picture of your life where options come into view, resources become visible, and even hope shows up in the larger view of your mind's eye. Try learning to appreciate how overcoming obstacles can draw out the better parts of yourself!

Engaging problems in my life has definitely made me a smarter woman. I have become much more strategic. After resolving each dilemma in life, I have become more equipped and experienced to be an example for others. I have gained wisdom to encourage others after facing each test. The more I go through, the more I grow through. Because of these truths, I view problems differently as I have learned to appreciate the benefits of hardships.

Change Your Response

After you change the way you view problems, you must change the way you respond to problems. This is where you begin to find opportunities to change your actions from prior responses you had that were ineffective.

In the worst of times, be a solution finder and not a problem finder. Do you know people that can find a problem many miles away but can't see a solution sitting on the tip of their nose? Are you that person?

Instead, you have to be intentional about finding ways to resolve a problem.

I have conditioned myself to respond to dilemmas from a position of power. It is a skill that I have sharpened by force and through repetition. Each day I have an opportunity to practice taking a power position against any attack. Whether a problem is major or minor, simple or complex, I take the same stance. I become a solver. I don't waste any time rehearsing the specifics of the problem because that is less time for me to strategize, and it delays my exit date.

Here is an example of a recurring issue I face since I drive almost three hours a day for work-related purposes. Picture me rolling down I-35 and seeing my engine and/or tire light come on an hour away from my destination. I am not at all comfortable with vehicle maintenance so this gives me anxiety. It may not be a problem of significance for others but it causes me to worry, so I have to begin my immediate transition from problem finder to solution finder.

I immediately begin encouraging myself. I tell myself that I will make it to the next car service station, or I will call for help from my husband or friends; if no one is available I will pull into a gas station and ask for help from a stranger. If that doesn't work, I will call an Uber driver. If I have no friends, no family, no Uber, no money, I will thank God I have legs and I will walk until I come up with my next strategy.

I also decide what I will not do. I will not be defeated. I will not be discouraged. I will not lose hope. I will not panic. That is a relatively minor problem but it illustrates my point that no matter what the obstacle, choose to find solutions and stop focusing on the details of the problem. Define options and dictate the rules of engagement as to what you will and will not do during the crisis. This change of behavior will propel you into a more abundant way of living as you will find yourself being more productive bettering your current problematic positions in life.

⤜ ⤜ ⤜

Of course, there are more traumatic circumstances that we all are dealing with. You may be experiencing a situation where you would love to begin to problem solve, but you do not even know where to start. This was me in the initial stages of my business venture. I was a young, pessimistic, relationally challenged and recently divorced single mother in my twenties with a new law firm solely in my hands. I also had no business experience. I did not have a clue how to manage business or people, and I only had a couple of years of experience practicing law.

I joined a law firm with two very experienced and prestigious partners in the community, an accomplished paralegal, and a legal secretary. I left a lucrative position with a guaranteed salary at a law firm, at the same time as divorcing, and I joined this partnership with the hopes of having a supportive launch into private practice being undergirded by the other established attorneys.

Within the first year of this venture, one of my partners became a judge and left the firm. This was a moment of celebration with a tinge of anxiety for me as now it was just myself and one other partner.

Within days of my first partner leaving to become a judge, the second partner told me he was not confident I would have enough business to support the overhead of the firm, therefore, he was also leaving. Not only was he leaving, but he was taking the office equipment and furniture with him because it belonged to him. I had little to nothing left of the offices when he moved.

Now it was myself, one paralegal, and the legal secretary who came with me. Within days of the second partner leaving, the experienced paralegal who had been working with the other two attorneys for years informed me that she was leaving the field and going into teaching, which was a nice way of her saying she needed to find other employment because the ship was sinking from her perspective. That left me and the legal secretary, along with all of the overhead of a law firm, all of the pressures of a business in my hands, and all of the challenges of single parenting resting on my shoulders.

I was beginning to lose confidence but I tried to encourage myself as I knew that I had to work twice as hard to produce the income to support all of the overhead alone that I once split with two other lucrative attorneys. I kept hope alive, as I still had one person left, my loyal legal secretary; and together we could do it.

Then there came the next blow. She came into my office in tears and informed me that her husband received orders to Alaska. That was it. There was no one left. In an office that was filled with attorneys, staff, support, income, clients, and business knowledge, there was only myself remaining. I cried. For a literal minute, I thought I failed. I rehearsed all of the problems to myself. I don't know to prepare any of the files for court. I don't know how to do payroll or QuickBooks. I don't know how to use the computer software for legal drafting. I don't know where to get new office furniture and so on and so forth.

I went home and took care of my daughter. The next morning, I went in to work and I walked from my office to the front desk where the legal secretary used to sit. I sat there and I started answering phones. I was smart enough to know that the most important thing to do now to feed my daughter was to keep the phones on and answer them, and try to bring clients in to hire me.

To my disappointment, the first phone call was not a new client but rather a paralegal from another office contacting me on a case we already had together. During the conversation, I began to think and pray, and the Holy Spirit gave me an idea—ask for help! I asked her if she knew anyone that could help me with paralegal work and she offered to work with me. I offered her a job right there on the phone. I decided in that moment that I would not be a victim and I had no time to sulk or shrink back from my commitment.

I was a business owner and I now own my own firm, and it is what I make of it. I knew I was alone but I would rebuild it from the ground with help. After the paralegal came, I was contacted by two attorneys that needed office space, so I rented my former partner's offices out to them and began to earn another source of income. That was the road to recovery. That was thirteen years ago and my business has become an abundant source of provision and joy.

Again, start with deciding that you are no longer subject to your problems but they are subject to you. Take whatever control you can in the moment, using all of your resources to put yourself in a position to begin to solve the problem. If it is a circumstance that you find yourself struggling to tackle alone, then enlist help.

Change Your Company

Change who you choose to engage about problems. During times like these you find out that you need help from other people. If you are fortunate, you have at least one person with wisdom that you can call to help you begin to problem solve. Not the person to sulk with you and add negativity. Not the person who listens to you and then shares their problems. Not the person that is too emotionally or financially invested to be a sober-minded unbiased advisor.

Ask yourself a few questions about the person before you submit yourself to their conversation and influence. Is this person optimistic? Is this person discreet? Does this person have a reputation for encouraging and being helpful to me in the past? After I talk to this person have I gained a better perspective or insight on the issue than I had before?

If you are a person with little to no support system, or in relationship with people who do not have the ability or capacity to advise you, then you have to find another resource. Remember, you began with deciding you are going to solve the problem so this obstacle of little resources or support has to be overcome as well.

You may need to go to the bookstore and read on the issue. You may need to make an appointment with a spiritual advisor in a nearby church or a counselor in your area. You may even need to go on Facebook and send a stranger a message asking for help.

You may think I'm being unrealistic but I am telling you what works. Be aggressive. This is how I met one of my closest friends. She contacted me on Facebook through messenger because she thought I was a Christian who prayed, and she wanted prayer for her anxiety, depression and high blood pressure.

Think outside of the box. There is always another option when you are ready to improve the quality of your life. My life gets better and better as I become a better problem solver. I have decided that every problem has a solution in which I play the starring role.

Changing the defeating parts of your mind, your heart, and your actions will place you in the proper position to receive and enjoy all that your abundant life has to offer you. Say this out loud, "The Abundant Life Starring Me!" Now that has a ring to it!

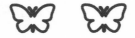

Chapter Three

Moving Forward

by Nicola Myers Gardere

> *I've learned that people will forget what you said, people will forget what you did, but people will never forget how you made them feel.*
>
> Maya Angelou

My usual get up and let's go attitude was clouded this morning with thoughts of the divorce proceedings that would be underway at 10:00 a.m. Getting the boys ready for day care and school seemed like a chore. My arms and legs were not cooperating with my brain, and a few times I felt like my heart was racing a thousand beats per minute.

In an effort not to transfer what I was feeling to the boys, I turned the TV to one of their favorite cartoons, or what I thought was their favorite cartoon at that moment. After dropping the kids off at school, I felt a loneliness rush over me like none I had felt before. I felt I was losing control and failing my children.

How could things change so quickly? How could someone else determine this was not working? I thought it was a partnership, I thought I had a say in how my family structure remained. The reality of the divorce proceedings that were scheduled for my day spoke otherwise. This is what he wanted and there was nothing I could do about it.

Anxiety in a man's heart weighs it down. But a good (encouraging) word makes it glad. [Proverbs 12:25, AMP]

Questions flooded my mind. My parents have been married for 52 years and continue to love and support each other despite any mitigating circumstances they have faced. Why does this not apply in my situation?

As I drove to work, I felt lost and helpless. Emotion after emotion washed over me. I remember crying out to God asking, "What have I done to be in this situation?" I was a good wife and the best mother to my children. I felt I let my parents and siblings down, who have managed to exist in successful marriages. I listened to my parents and did everything in my power to make them proud. They set an incredible example for us to follow, they showed us what a healthy marriage looked like, what resilience is and how to make it through.

Regardless of how many similarities existed, I felt I failed myself, my children and my family. This was just a snippet of the thoughts that raced through my mind. I was devastated, anxious, confused, angry, hurt and betrayed. I knew I had to get myself together and be strong. I tried to encourage myself and snap out of the darkness engulfing me, but I was unable to think rationally or logically.

Somehow, I got myself to work that morning. As I stood in front of an eager class of elementary students ready to apply and make connections through the lesson I had prepared for them, I watched the clock slowly tick its way to 10:00 a.m. I heard every second tick on the classroom clock, with every tick I felt fear tighten around my heart. I looked around and my students were engaged and working in collaborative groups. That time stood out to me because that's the time I was scheduled to appear in court.

I made a decision not to go to court because in my mind, it was an indication to me that I wanted to be a part of the dissolution of my marriage—of my life as I had known it. Though I wouldn't be physically present in the court room, I exerted what control I had in this life changing event by ensuring that the contents of that yellow envelope and everything to do with the well-being of my children were agreed upon. I was the custodial parent and that's all that mattered to me.

The hands of the clock landed on 10:00 a.m. and almost like the training bombs I hear in the mornings living next to a military base, it felt like an explosion and everything stopped. The clock stopped and so did my heart, well at least it felt like my heart stopped. My teacher assistant was not aware of what was taking place. I am very private in my personal life. I don't like being judged or letting anyone get close enough to me to get into my life.

I wish someone knew what I was going through at that point. I needed a hug and no one knew my life was falling apart. What if I fainted under the pressure of what was going on? What if I just lost it? I didn't want to scare my students, but everything seemed out of control. Maybe I should have stayed home today. Maybe I still had time to leave—all sorts of thoughts raced through my mind and then it hit me. I am divorced!

Be still and know that I am God. I will be exalted among the nations, I will be exalted in the earth. [Psalm 46:10 NIV]

I am no longer a wife, and my kids will only have one parent in the home. I can't imagine what that will be like. My dad is still in my life and at home. How will they know the feeling of growing up in a two-parent household?

This was the best time to ask my teacher's assistant to take over the class. I had to get away in a private space. Shaking like a leaf, legs trembling, my heart palpating, I made my way to the bathroom and found some relief as I wretched my guts out. But, this was no time to collapse, I had to compose myself in order to make it through the day.

My Aunt Pat always used to remind me to be still and let God take care of me. Despite what was going on around me, she would have expected me to pull myself together and know that God was going to work it out. I diligently, if not robotically, fixed my makeup, slapped on a fake smile and walked back to my classroom. My head knew God was in control but, more importantly, I had to find a way to believe and trust Him so my heart could heal.

The bell eventually rang and to everyone else it signified class change, but it was so much more for me, my life as I had known it was gone. Change was here whether or not I wanted it. As the students filed out of the classroom I fought back tears at the irony of the parallels.

>||> >||> >||>

My life has never been the same since my divorce. I worked harder than any parent I knew to ensure my kids had a good life. I ensured they were enrolled in every sport, every season. I was present for every practice even through pain and sickness.

I am a chronic migraine sufferer, I recall one of many practice events and the agony I went through. My older son had a soccer practice on the fields of Ellison High School, little did I know that many years later he would graduate from that same high school and play on the same field he practiced on as a little boy.

That day, I was in a full blown migraine episode and my head felt as if it were going to explode. My son told me, "Mom, it's ok for us to miss practice." I told him, "You forge through any situation life presents, we are going to your practice."

I remembered my mom's words, "Dear God, my cup runneth over." There are many ways this may be interpreted. Some may interpret this as an overflowing of blessings. However, mom's interpretation was connected to her being overwhelmed and her acknowledgement that she couldn't take any more on top of what she was faced with. I chose to attach mom's interpretation in this situation.

In the same breath, I clung to another phrase that she would always follow up with, "This too shall pass." What my mom did was acknowledge her present circumstance but found a way to find hope. This is the silent resiliency she taught us. Despite what you are faced with, there is a light at the end of the tunnel.

In a two-parent household, I would imagine, this is the time the other parent would take the kids to practice but, TAG, I was both parents! I packed two bags of ice and grabbed my pillow. As my son practiced, I held an ice pack to my forehead and one on the back of my neck. I laid on the pillow and occasionally peered up to catch a play.

The kids and I talked after every practice and I had to capture something to engage and be a part of the conversation on the ride home. At one point, I recall stopping to open the door to throw up from the nausea that accompanied every migraine episode. I got used to pushing through the pain, making every effort to support my children in what I call an unusual situation.

It would have been easy to just lay in the bed and writhe in pain and allow myself to wallow in my circumstances, but God gave me a fighting spirit and I had to trust that He would see me through. I could have taken the easy way out and taken my prescription medication, but that would have rendered me unable to drive.

Now that practice was over, homework done, dinner done, and everyone bathed and in bed, I took my medication and went to sleep. I would feel better eventually, but my kids were my priority. It was my duty to ensure they participated and had a full life experience growing up.

Lessons from growing up in a family of God fearing grandparents always seem to bubble up. I kept hearing my grandma's voice. "Weeping may endure for a night but joy cometh in the morning." (Psalm 30:5). At the end of the day, the boys had a great soccer practice, I felt satisfied because I did not allow my circumstances to determine how our day ended.

I cried out at night when the lights went out and I was alone. I was terrified. What if I failed my children? I am all they have. Why did God allow this to happen to me? If my kids were unsuccessful in life, it would be a result of my failure to prepare them for life. This was a huge responsibility, one that kept me up on many nights.

On days when my mom was frustrated with situations presented to her, I remembered she would always sigh and say, "God does not give me more that I can bear." I wondered if what I was feeling was the feeling she experienced? The darkness? The despair? The uncertainty? My parents didn't prepare me for divorce because in our family, despite what you are faced with, you work through it. Weeping may last a night, but joy comes in the morning. I asked God for the joy-filled days, the joy in the morning. I cried going to bed and waking up in the mornings. This was too much for me to handle.

>₪ >₪ >₪

A man's heart plans his way, but the Lord directs his steps. [Proverbs 16:9 NKJV]

My ex-husband and I both decided to stay in Central Texas to give the boys some sense of normalcy in what I thought was an abnormal situation. On the weekends they were with their dad, it gave me a break to catch up on my sleep and volunteer in the community. Despite my circumstances, I am a servant leader and was taught by my grandmother that serving in the house of the Lord and community was important.

As the years went by and we adjusted to a life without the other parent in the home, I decided I had to change my career path. I went back to college and earned two more degrees: Bachelors of Science in Human Services Management, a Master's degree in English Language Arts/Curriculum & Instruction, and a Principal certification K-12th grade.

With age comes more demands to participate in sports on a different level. Participating in activities outside the parks and recreation was expensive and time consuming. My older son wrestled with the high school and the Mat Katz on Fort Hood, and my younger son played basketball for the high school and with various Amateur Athletic Union (AAU) teams. The practices were regular and sometimes further away from the home.

It was time to increase my value and make myself more marketable. The challenge of going back to college came with my kids at home. This meant sacrificing long nights and weekends to meet all the demands. I recall going to bed at 3am after writing long papers, and my alarm going off at 6am to get the day started. Reaching over to snooze the alarm was not an option. Getting up and facing another day and being purposeful and productive was my purpose.

I am a naturalized Canadian citizen living in Texas. Sometimes, I felt alone in Texas. However, I made the decision to stay there to ensure the boys were around their dad, even if that meant a few days, or even hours, on the weekend. There were times when that did not happen, and I didn't question why I stayed, but at the end of the day I relied on the word of God to carry me through and erased the questions.

>⧫ >⧫ >⧫

A few months prior to the divorce my then mother-in-law came to live with us. Soon after arriving she was diagnosed with cancer and was facing a battle of her own. That rocked the family but we had a strong bond and decided to fight our battles together. Her words of comfort resonated with me on some of my darkest days when I could not see the light. I started relying on her strength even in her weakest moments.

I know thy works: behold, I have set before thee an open door, and no man can shut it: for thou hast a little strength, and hast kept My word, and has not denied My name. [Revelations 3:8 KJV]

Ave Maria can be heard coming from the bedroom down the hallway or an old hymn being sang by the most beautiful voice one could imagine. My younger son even mimicked the words and my older son repeated her prayers. She was a praying woman, a God-fearing woman and a loving grandma who gave of herself to stay with us after the divorce. On any given Sunday my pastor talked of 'door openers'. The doors God had opened for us could not be closed by anyone. My mother-in-law became one of my sources of strength and I was determined to allow God to use us to carry each other.

I prayed for God to give me the courage and strength to face the unknown. Little did I know that my dearest friend who lay in the next room battling cancer would become my angel. Yes, my mother-in-law decided to stay with me to help see me and the boys through the effects of the divorce from her son.

Most would question such a pairing, most thought she was the lucky one. But no, the boys and I were the lucky ones. See, what most don't know or cannot begin to understand is that she was sent by God. She showed me how to be still and know that God was in charge and would do amazing things in my life if I just trust that He would.

Having gone through medical school years prior, my mother-in-law reminded me that a nosebleed would be ok. When my older son had a gel-like substance covering his eyes due to severe allergies, she told me it would be ok, exactly what the diagnosis would be, and how the doctors would treat it. I learned to listen to wisdom. She was the gentle spirit God sent down the hallway to help carry me though my anxiety when I thought everything was the end to the world.

My mother-in-law became my best friend, my support, my other mother and one of the best grandmothers my boys could ever ask for. She loved us and she took care of us. Despite the loss (divorce) that I was faced with, she reminded me to fight though the pain, to be strong and never let my faith waver despite my circumstances. Yes, cancer was here and we prayed for her strength and the disease to let go of her body.

As I sit here and document the experiences, I miss her terribly. Going through my darkest moments or what I thought was my darkest moments was a set up for a comeback. Most people that have heard of our story compared our connection to Ruth and Naomi in the Bible. I researched and read the story to become familiar with it.

While there were many parallels to our situation, one that was clear to me was that she was helping me more that I could ever imagine. We often joked that my Boaz was coming. When favorable things occur in my life and that of my children, I always whisper a quiet thank you to my mother-in-law. She told me God would bless and take care of me for the love and compassion I showed her. I was given an assignment and I asked God to give me the strength to fulfill His will. Give me the energy when I felt weary and also to comfort me at night when I was overwhelmed.

As I went through the fight of her life with her, I would set a bath schedule for her just like I did the boys, spoon fed her, dressed her, brushed her teeth and massaged her feet as I applied lotion. I reassured her that I would never ever leave her. Despite what she faced and what her body was going through, she found the strength to encourage me and smile. She refused to let cancer or pain steal her joy or praise.

I started looking at my situation through different lens and strangely thanked God for the test. I knew that despite my current situation, I must praise God and find a way to smile. Most nights, the boys and I would stay in her room talking and laughing until we all fell asleep. I miss my mother-in-law, she was my rock though my hardest years, she made a bright light shine into situations where all I saw was darkness.

And Ruth said, intreat me not to leave thee, or to return from following after thee: for wither thou goest, I will go; and where thou lodgest, I will lodge: thy people shall be my people, and thy God my God. [Ruth 1:16 KJV]

Most questioned why five years after my divorce from her son we lived together. What most don't understand when God has placed people in your life and set up the situation, you simply remain obedient and let God do what He said He would do. Years after we made it through cancer, came dementia, yet another test. That struggle was real. However, despite memory loss and eventually moving her to a nursing home, the one person that would create a calmness around me that I couldn't explain while in Texas, was my angel, my mother-in-law.

Despite trials and tribulations, as my sons went through the teen age years and when my nerves were on edge, driving to the nursing home and laying in her bed filled me with a safe and calm feeling like none other. On many occasions when I went to visit her, she would not be in her room because she wandered somewhere else and sometimes was found laying in someone else's bed. As soon as I showed up, her entire face would glow. I saw a light in her that neither cancer nor dementia silenced. We would walk back to her bed and lay down together. As she laid closest to the wall, she would occasionally reach her hand back and pat me. Something I could still feel today, the most reassuring touch to remind me to be still and trust God.

See, divorce, cancer, and dementia made our bond stronger. As I sat in the nursing home alone with her waiting for the coroner to pick her body up, she looked as if she was sleeping. I cried and asked God to let the seeds she planted in me carry me through. As I talked to her, I felt her warmth even though her spirit was gone, I could feel the love. I smiled through my tears, she had fought a great fight and God saw fit to take her. I didn't question God, instead I thanked Him for giving her to us.

I still think of her on a daily basis and miss her presence deeply. She still carries me through with her words of comfort. Despite being gone to be with the Lord, she planted seeds in us that will never die. Who would have known that a divorce from her son would create a lasting friendship that cancer, dementia nor death could break? The boys and I all learned how to be still and know that God was in control.

>⧐ >⧐ >⧐

Today, my ex-husband and I are friends, we raised out boys together from the day of our divorce. There were years when I was angry and upset with him especially when my sons had to deal with the pain that came with the divorce and his lack of presence for a couple years. We are all recovering and I thank God for carving out my path and for allowing us to continue to raise our sons 19 years after divorce. My kids are still finding that peace of forgiveness, but on a daily basis their dad is showing them that he is there and does not plan on leaving any time soon.

>⧐ >⧐ >⧐

As I write this, I am a year away from completing my Doctorate Degree in Educational Leadership. Resilience and peace is connected and provided me with the strength and determination I needed to see through the days I thought were the darkest, and to show my kids what success looks like.

Through my divorce and the death of my mother-in-law, I learned how to adapt in the face of adversity.

I continue to bounce back despite everything that the devil meant to destroy me. The stress and traumatic experiences have shaped who I have become today.

With a fiery granddaughter and two adult children, one with a college degree in Information Systems Technology, and my other son currently a sophomore in college pursuing a course of study leading to sports medicine. I am the face of resiliency and will overcome anything that is set in front of me.

Many would ask, how did you do it? I encourage you to seek out support groups if you don't have anyone around you that can pour positivity and encouragement into you daily. Ensuring that your confidante is able to add value to you and lift you up is important to your emotional well-being and growth.

As I examined my situation, I quickly became aware that in order to sustain a one parent household and remain in the home instead of working several jobs, I made the decision to go back to school and further my education. Changing your mindset and have clear goals you want to achieve will help you on the days when you feel you have nothing left to give. Working with the end in mind carried me through. In my current situation I have created a vision board. The goal is to keep moving forward. Keep advancing and the sky will be the limit.

Burnout is sure to creep up on you sometimes. I learned to value the weekends my kids were with their dad, and made a conscious effort to sleep in and go to the gym. Being physically and emotionally fit created the gateway that I needed to stay on track and recharge.

With my family living in Canada, I became creative with my vacations and the boys were grateful for the extra time with their cousins. My parents and sisters took turns flying in to town to pick the boys up a week before I joined them. This gave me additional free time to close out each semester in school and do big projects around the house. Cleaning out closets and donating items to Goodwill was an actual job with young kids in the house.

One of the most challenging yet rewarding tasks was teaching the boys not to hold animosity or anger towards their dad. We spent time together with the boys teaching them how to get along and respect their parents regardless of the separation or divorce.

As a grandmother to an adoring granddaughter, my older son shared with me that he has no clue how I was able to maintain everything I did without showing anger towards his dad. I taught my kids to love, but in doing so I had to show them *how*. As I type this, their dad and I continue to have dinner with them or breakfast when everyone is in town, and of course our little addition is at the table speaking nonstop. She adores her grandparents because now we have to teach her how to love despite divorce and separation.

One of my favorite quotes that currently sits over my desk reminds me to never stop moving forward regardless of what I am faced with. Dr. Martin Luther King, Jr. once said, "If you can't fly then run. You can't run then walk. If you can't walk then crawl, but whatever you do, you have to keep moving forward."

Chapter four

God is With Her

by Brigette Marie

> *Your destiny isn't determined on their decision to stay in your life. If people want to walk out of your life, let them walk.*
>
> Bishop T.D. Jakes

She grew up admiring a well-known actress most knew as Shirley Temple, with just as much heart and love for all—welcoming of all people, no matter their gender, race or socioeconomic status. As a young child, she had confidence, independence, and had a knack for not conforming to the norms of her surroundings.

As her grandparents would notice, she was adorable and witty. Additionally, she always knew the direction she would go in life, and really had no idea how she was going to get there but knew, without a doubt, she would reach her dreams. She never really had it easy growing up—forcing her to rise above challenging times. She was faced with alcoholism, physical and emotional abuse, and instability throughout her upbringing. How did this impact her? How did she cope?

Around the age of eight, the man she loved most in life threatened to kill her. She experienced divorce multiple times as her parents sought to find happiness in the love another could give them. The day her brother was diagnosed with cerebral palsy, she knew that she would one day be a nurse.

Throughout her teenage and adolescent years, she was known by many, but called only a few her friends. She remembered making vows to herself that she would not be an alcoholic; she would not be addicted to drugs; she would not be abusive to her children and they would be the center of her life; she would marry once and not be another statistic in divorce. As her siblings and many of the youth in her era experimented with things like sex, drugs, and alcohol, she stayed focused—not because people in her life directed her to, but because it truly was who she was. She had an inner strength that was different from so many of her family because "God is within her, she will not fail."

Hello there, my name is Brigette Marie. I am a forty-one-year-old single woman, mother, daughter, friend, sister, veteran and nurse. I spent the first nine years of my life in Chicago, Illinois and the next nine in Northern Arizona. I then joined the United States Army, where I served for almost 11 years.

While I served, I met and married a man who I believed was the absolute love of my life. That decision produced my three phenomenal sons, who make me a better person every day; they truly are my pride and joy. Throughout my story, I will elaborate on what I thought was the weakest moment in my life that ultimately revealed the strength that was hidden deep within my spirit. In sharing, I hope to encourage you and push you to be better than you ever thought imaginable.

Although my worst moment was in the midst of divorce, you can apply the same actions and principles to any storm you face, to carry you through to your victory. No matter your age, learn to love yourself first, give yourself the attention you deserve, always strive to be all that you desire to be, and you WILL make it—it is ALL possible!

The Storm

As I stated before, I married the man of my dreams March 10, 2001. Truth be told, he really was. I am bold. I am opinionated. I am driven. I am stubborn. I am also a fireball. Although I handle chaos and stress in my chosen field of nursing well, in my upbringing, I learned that happiness was gained or lived only when others did what you asked them to and if they didn't, that action equaled a lack of love.

I learned that love was conditional. For instance, if I tell you "hey, take out the trash on your way out the door," and you didn't, that usually resulted in a screaming match, full blown anger from me. Like how hard is it to do what you are asked?

My husband was my polar-opposite. He was the calmness in our relationship. He was strength. He was patience. He was wisdom. He understood me. We met in the Army while stationed in Germany. I was in a relationship when we met, but he was persistent in his pursuit of me. The relationship I was in ended abruptly and he was there to pick up the pieces of my broken heart.

It is important to mention that the relationship ended abruptly because it was made known that he was a married man. It was easy to let him go because he was married, and I knew there was this other guy that had made his interest known to me so I would not be alone. Looking back, I realized that being alone was a fear I had but wasn't really mindful of at that time. It was that fear that allowed me to look past many of the warning signs that should have caused me to run in the other direction.

However, this new guy was there to make me feel immediately wanted again. He was there to keep me from feeling alone and give me attention that I was seeking—from the opposite sex that is. He was kind to me. He was gentle. He accepted my bubbly outgoing, loving spirit. He shared things with me that I still believe he had never shared with anyone, and I believe that we grew to know each other better than we knew ourselves.

The times I enjoyed most were simply laying on his lap as he ran his fingers through my hair and I fell asleep. His warmth. His touch. His smile. His simple presence. As a result of my fear of being alone and not being accepted caused me to dismiss the obvious warning signs I experienced in my relationship with him.

While in Germany, we had many break-ups but we always ended up back in each other's arms. There was never physical or verbal abuse. Our break-ups were ALWAYS due to his unfaithfulness. Remember I said I wasn't really fond of being alone right? So there you have it—he cheats, I get upset, break-up, he apologizes, I forgive, we get back together and the cycle is on repeat.

I never really had anyone waiting on me so if I took him back, I didn't have to be alone. I cannot say when it was that I made him the source of my happiness, but I did and as a result, I lost myself in the process. I dealt with choices that he made, that I really should not have, because I didn't want to lose him and be alone. He always smoothed talked his way out of it and/or apologized. I forgave him and took him back. Looking back, his unfaithfulness developed insecurities in myself that I held on to that I did not have growing up, or... maybe I did???

We were still in a relationship but had not married prior to me leaving Europe. About a month after my arrival to my next duty station, I found out that I was pregnant. I was so scared but also excited, and so was he. As I learned growing up to face my fears, he revealed that he didn't. Our relationship seemed more distant than ever really. Although he was now out of the Army, he did not join me in Oklahoma but instead lived on the East coast with his family. He arrived one week before our first son was born and left one week after his birth, and again I was alone.

Shortly after he left, I received a message from his girlfriend stating, "How can you love him and you cheated on him? He said it isn't even his baby!" I had not cheated on him but that was the lie he told her. I was crushed. He denied to this woman his child whom he named after him. How could he do such a thing? I cussed him out. I cussed her out. (Don't judge me, you know you would have had some select words as well.)

Needless to say, that was the end of that relationship for me... or not.

Six months after my first son's birth, I re-enlisted in the military to take advantage of the opportunity for the Army to train me to be a nurse. While I was in training, my first-born son went to live with my father and my step-mother for six months, and then joined me then in Fort Gordon, Georgia. During the next two years, I was in and out of three to four relationships.

Again, I was never without some type of companion but nothing ever really serious. I kept my distance from this word "love". While I was in Georgia, my child's father came to me and said he wanted me back and wanted our family to work. Although I had been without him for so long at that point, my heart truly wanted the same and we married March 10, 2001. That was the beginning of six years of marital infidelity.

There were many times I felt shamed, foolish and belittled. We had mutual friends, who I later learned he told that I knew about his extra relationships and that I was okay with them. There were many moments of happiness as well, but six years later our marriage ended in divorce.

We went down the emotional roller coaster in our marriage as well. I'd find out he was unfaithful. I'd be hurt. I'd decide to forgive and stay. Things were good. It'd happen again. Another repeat cycle. I feel the need to add that there were at least two times that I decided "I'm just gonna get even. I'll show him that he is not my all." Although temporarily satisfying, it was just that, temporary because we always ended up back together.

At the moment of our divorce, I was getting out of the United States Army, I had two sons, ages 5 and 8 years old, I was pregnant, without a job and without a husband. I was devastated. I spent endless hours and months crying in bed. I would go days without showering. Every decision I made was focused on his happiness. I gave everything I was to him. My purpose in life was to make him happy. How could he not love me back? What was wrong with me? I supported him. I encouraged him. I believed in him. I loved him. But did I? Did I really love him or did I just not love myself?

I remember sitting on the cold concrete of my driveway asking him to tell me why he couldn't love me the way I loved him. His response was, "There is nothing wrong with you, it's me." I learned that this was only half true. How could I have loved him when I lost the ability to love myself? Who was I? Did I know my worth? When did I begin to lose my self-worth? Did I ever love me? That was the beginning of my journey to becoming all that God, my children and the world needed me to be.

You Are a Queen – Trust Your King

In the opening paragraph, I explained who I was as a little girl and all that I had planned in store for my life. The "she" was me. I was full of life and hopes and I had declared that I would not be a statistic in the world of divorce. I struggled greatly with that decision. So much so that I dealt with infidelity for many years before deciding to end my marriage. I was lost and confused.

My first advice to you is to ALWAYS seek wise counsel before you make life changing decisions. Here is what my battle was about. I believe in generational curses. I believe that what happens in the generation before you, that resulted in a failure of a successful outcome, will come to visit the following generation. With that being said, I had a decision to make. Do I continue to allow divorce or infidelity to reign in my generations to come? At that point, I had three sons, if I stayed in a marriage that was full of unfaithfulness by either spouse, what would I be teaching them? How am I teaching them to treat the woman they love? In divorce, am I teaching them to give up?

Both of my parents divorced twice and remarried a third time. As a result, I went through the roller coaster of emotions as a child, and I wanted to shield them from that, but was I? Were they not already experiencing some of the roller coaster of emotions that their dad and I were acting on? I battled for years with that decision to divorce him. I was confused and did not know which way to turn. As a result, I sought out counsel from my spiritual mother. She reminded me that God does not intend for us to be unhappy. She never told me directly, "You need to get a divorce."

What she did was went to her office and brought back colorful copies of a few, "Love Letters from Your King" and read them to me. (To this day, they are still framed and hung on my home walls as reminders of His love for me.) As she had me read them, tears began to flow like Niagara Falls as the words pierced my soul.

"My Princess… You're Never Alone. You never need to hold on to anyone out of fear of being alone. My precious princess. I am with you wherever you are. I am the friend who walks in when the world walks out. I created you to have strong relationships, My love, and I see your desire to be close to someone. If you will seek Me first and come to Me with your wants and needs, I will choose your friends for you. I also will bless those friendships abundantly. Don't settle for less than My best just to fill your schedule with people to see and places to go. I want to reach you with the reality of My presence in you first, and then you will be ready for real relationships that are orchestrated by Me." – His Princess: Love Letters from Your King by Sheri Rose Shepherd[1]

"My Princess… Guard Your Heart. If I were to hand you a fragile, newborn baby girl, I know that you would protect her with your life. Your arms would be strong, your feet sure, and your eyes ever watchful. Be careful, My trusted one! For I have placed something just as precious and delicate within you. It is your heart… your very life! Treasure it. Protect it. Watch over it with all your strength. For the world and all its pleasures are like kidnappers who will stop at nothing to steal your heart away from Me and destroy it. I want what is best for you, My treasured one, and although you sometimes feel that the sinful pleasures of this world don't seem harmful, they will separate you from ME. Just as a newborn is helpless without loving care, you also will suffer if your heart is taken from Me. So, I'm asking you to guard your heart and cling to Me, the Source of your life." – His Princess: Love Letters from Your King by Sheri Rose Shepherd[1]

Fear had taken over me up until that point. Much like my parents, I was in fear of being alone. I didn't want to parent alone. I did not want to be alone. I didn't want to go through life alone. But those, and a few other letters, penetrated my heart and gave me courage to make the decision I had struggled for years to make.

>#> >#> >#>

I have now been single for ten years. God has never let me down. I have never gone without. I had to learn to trust someone I couldn't see which wasn't easy. I couldn't in general trust people that I could see, and now God was calling me to trust Him. Everyday has not been easy but His promises to me are just that and He will not and has not lied or forsaken me.

I highly recommend that you get a copy of the book by Sheri Rose Shepherd mentioned above. It has close to 100 letters from God to you – His princess. And when life is trying to get the best of you, read your King's letter to you to lift you up and push you to keep walking through your storm. It will even help you to encourage your daughters as they face their day-to-day challenges in their lives as well.

Building Your Self-Esteem

So now that I have this revelation that I needed to trust God, what now? Just because I knew that I needed to leave the damaging relationship that I was in, it didn't make all my insecurities that had surfaced go away. For about four years after my divorce, I went back and forth with my ex-husband, still trying to keep hold of his "love". He was familiar. He was what I knew. He was the life I had learned to adjust to. Like a physically abused woman going back to an abusive relationship. Like a drug addict or alcoholic back sliding to deal with life stressors as if it ever really made the problems go away. It was a cycle I continued to live year after year after year.

How do I get free? How do I build from here? What was that situation teaching me? What I knew was that I needed to find myself again.

Who am I? What am I worth? What is my purpose? I had to take ownership of my happiness but how? As I dug deeper and deeper into "how did I get here" and "what am I supposed to learn from this", I began to realize that when I started to change the way I looked at these things or my situation, the things I saw in the situation began to change.

Here is what I mean. Throughout the process of divorce and the four years following, I looked at who my husband was and what he did to hurt me. As time went on, I decided to focus on myself and what my role was in the situation. As I did that, I began to focus on what I could change and that was myself. I am not saying that it was my "fault" for his infidelity. I am saying I played the biggest role in my choice to stay and live with the unfaithfulness as well as the emotions I had packed up and carried with me daily.

At that point, I had hit my "rock bottom". I was lost. I needed to find myself. I needed to take responsibility for myself and my behavior within that failed relationship. By responsibility, I mean response–able; I am able to be in control of the response I have and I have the ability to choose what that response will be.

So many times, in life, we want to look at someone else and blame others for what we are experiencing. For so long, my behavior was a product of the conditions I was experiencing and my feelings that were produced within that relationship. We have the responsibility to decide how any situation will affect us. In my divorce, I had control over whether or not I would allow him to have control over my decisions. Quite honestly, it was MY self-doubt that crept in and caused me to make decisions that ultimately caused me to lose myself in the relationship. I had to decide to change my response to his actions and be in control of my behavior.

I always had a choice and I chose to stay. He NEVER said, "You need to make me happy." That was all my doing and I have learned that I am NOT in control of anybody else's happiness except for my own. That little girl had values that she lost somewhere along the way. I decided that my behaviors would now be a product of decisions made based on the values, my values, that I held to be true to me so long ago. I began to live my life for me.

At that point, I literally cut off the outside noise of the world and focused on myself. I listened to seminars, read books, and attended women's conferences that helped build who I was, beginning with a solid foundation.

One of the most life changing audios that I listened to was a series from Christine Martin titled "Creating a Positive Self-Image: Celebrating the Uniqueness of You!"[2] The series begins by reminding me that I am fearfully and wonderfully made in His image and likeness (Psalm 139:14). That I am unique, different from any other woman out there—I wasn't called to be like anyone else but me. It taught me to be in control of me and taught me that I am in no way in control or responsible for others' happiness except my own.

I then made little changes daily to renew my mind and reprogram my mental thinking through speaking positive confessions over my life. What I ultimately learned is that without my permission, no one can make me feel inferior or less than. The same holds true for you.

Additionally, I read a book titled, "Your Divine Fingerprint: The Force That Makes YOU Unstoppable" by Keith Craft.[3] Through reading this book, I learned that I, which also means that YOU, have the power to decide how any moment in our life will affect us. It explains that there is a process that we all go through that produces a result that cannot be produced any other way.

For instance, in algebra, say that there is an equation like $2x+8=20$. There is only one answer for "x" in order for this equation result to be 8. "X" will produce a result that cannot be produced any other way. Keith Craft calls this our "X" factor.

With God, He is always trying to teach and grow us. In teaching us, there is a path that we will need to take to get us to the destination He wants us to get to. It is our "X" factor; it is the situation that will produce the outcome God wants in the development of who we need to be. It is unique, just like you.

Why am I sharing this? Because I want you to decide to never grow weary in any situation that life deals you. Know that there is a reason and a purpose that will produce who you need to be. There is so much more that we need to learn and explore about ourselves. Much like your fingerprint is unique to who you are, your "X" factor is unique as well and is instrumental in your unique journey.

How to Guard Your Heart

How do I guard my heart in order to keep my happiness in check? Boundaries. If you are anything like me, you, too, have a problem telling people no because you are loving and giving. Maybe, like myself, you are a people pleaser. Although you can handle conflict, it is surely not your first choice in how you handle people or differences so you will do what you deem necessary to keep peace.

The problem I have found with this logic is that, eventually, as we please others, and things are not returned or our actions aren't viewed as appreciated, we feel frustrated, neglected, ignored, walked over, etc. Suddenly we are angry, bitter, hurt, short-tempered, experience feelings of guilt, loss of love, connection or approval and ultimately unhappy. And why? Because we did not take the time to set boundaries for our lives. So often we secretly endure the pain of the other person's irresponsibility as opposed to letting them know how their decisions affect us because we did not take the time to set boundaries for our lives.

What exactly is a boundary? It is a line that marks limits off an area. Your personal boundaries help to identify who you are. You need to place boundaries on who can touch you and who cannot; who can speak into your life and who cannot; what actions of others you deem acceptable and which actions are not; when you will stay and when you will go. Identifying these types of boundaries that are important to you helps you to guard your heart.

Dr. Henry Cloud and Dr. John Townsend have written a book titled, "Boundaries."[4] In this book, they help to identify when to say 'yes' and how to say 'no' in a pursuit to take control of your life. They share that our boundaries need to be made visible and communicated to any person we come in contact with. If in our boundary setting, someone is unable to handle our boundary, it is okay to let them walk away or for us to walk away. Everyone is not intended to be a part of our life; the people that are meant to be in your life will stay.

You were created to be exactly who you are—a Queen. You are loved. You are worthy. You are beautiful. You are fearless. You are unstoppable. You are courageous. You are strength. You are intelligent. Your happiness should be the most important aspect of your life and is the one thing in an ever-changing world of which you have sole responsibility.

Do what you love. Be who you are naturally. Guard your heart. Set your boundaries. Don't allow others to change who you are. This is your life—live it. You are a phenomenal woman!

Chapter five

Conquering Depression

by Vannette P. Simmons

Trust yourself. Think for yourself. Act for yourself. Speak for yourself. Be yourself. Imitation is suicide.

Marva Collins

By the time I realized what was happening to me, the process had already been set in motion. Why had I woken up with tears in my eyes? Was I even awake? As I became aware of the bed I was lying in and the position of my body, I realized there was something in my hands. My fists were clenched tightly around my shirt. In my sleep, I had been crying and tearing at my clothes. Maybe it was all a bad dream. Maybe I dreamed that I got that call that would change our lives life forever.

As I type this, recalling that day still causes me quite a bit of anxiety. I was at work and I received a cryptic call from my brother-in-law who seldom called me. "Are you at home?" "How long will you be at work?" He asked. "I probably will be another hour or so, is everything ok," I responded. "Yeah, just call me when you get home," he said. "Okay" I was not sure what he had to tell me, but I could hear in his voice that something had happened.

As I pulled into my driveway a few hours later he called me again. "Hey, you have great timing, I just pulled in," I said. "What going on?" I asked. "Wayne passed," I heard my brother-in-law say on the other end of the line. "What?" I responded confused. "Passed where, passed what?" Wayne, was the childhood nickname of my estranged husband of 14 years.

Dwayne (Wayne) was a Captain in the United States Army, and he had recently returned from his third deployment overseas. At the time, I was living in our home in Killeen, Texas, and he was stationed in a different state. Every time he went on a deployment, he came back just a little different. It was as if he left parts of himself, the parts I knew and loved, somewhere else, yet returned with strange parts which did not agree with us. He physically looked like my husband, but bit by bit his personality had morphed into a different person.

Quite frankly, I became a different person as well. Each time he went away, I was a single parent once again for at least nine or more months at a time. I had learned to navigate being a full-time student while working a full-time job. I cared for our two very active pre-teen children. I made sure they got to and excelled in all of their academic and extra-curricular activities. Our social lives were very involved with activities such as Tae Kwon Do, gymnastics, dance, piano lessons, and whatever sport was in season. As a family, we also stayed active in our church. Unfortunately, three deployments later, our marriage was on a road that had been stripped, with wonder as to when it was going to be paved.

How did we even get on that road? When we met in college we talked about growing old together like Ossie Davis and Ruby Dee. We were inseparable in those early days. We often shared our dreams with each other of graduating from college, landing dream jobs, getting married, and planning a family. We were living our dream just as we had planned. Along the path we were paving, we seemed to have lost sight of each other.

I was still sitting in my car but I could barely breathe. Brother-in-law repeated himself but I could not really hear him anymore. Dwayne never explained that he was leaving, nor did he ever express any of those feelings. In fact, we spoke just the day before after I texted him a picture of our baby girl. It was the first amicable conversation we had had in a while. That alone caused a plethora of feelings. Despite all of the feelings of betrayal, maybe there was hope for us. So where did he go? My brother-in-law repeated himself slowly and carefully, "Wayne passed, Vannette. He passed." My heart sunk.

I could feel my face go numb and I could not hear anything else he said to me as I slowly came to realize what my brother-in-law had meant. I was sitting in our driveway, staring into one of the windows to our home. Realizing again that I had arrived home, our children were already watching me through that same window. I tried to look past them as I stared in disbelief. Our son, my husband's pride and joy, was twelve and his sister, the apple of her daddy's eye, was ten. What I was about to tell them was going to change their worlds forever. How was I supposed to go inside and tell them? Dwayne died. My husband, my college sweetheart and their father was gone. Forever? Forever.

≫⊩ ≫⊩ ≫⊩

As I mentioned earlier, my husband and I were estranged. Irreconcilable differences are what I remember the lawyer calling it. We separated in June and by the end of August he was gone. Forever gone. We were about to grieve who he used to be and who he was slowly becoming. Looking back at the whole situation now, it's like we lost him twice in such a short period of time. Although our relationship had spanned almost 20 years, it only took three months for our world to come totally undone. At the time that is what it felt like. That hurt was so deep and so huge I could not see a way out of it. How was everyone around me able to function? I wanted and needed the healing process to start to take place. I knew that grief had to run its course and that for each person there was no statute of limitations on how short or long that could be. There was also more going on than just grief of losing my longtime partner. There was the lingering feeling that somehow our relationship failed because I was not enough and now there was no way to talk things out.

Nevertheless, I also knew that I was a fixer. It is what I do. I make things right. I fix things and then we all move on and live happily ever after like in a sitcom. But in that situation, I did not want to do the work. The process ahead just seemed too messy. This messy work would cause me, cause us, our babies, our family to have to go to a dark place where I did not want to be.

Edward Hirsch, in his book, "Gabriel"[5], explains that when you lose someone you love, you are missing them and simultaneously longing for what you lost in yourself. He discusses that grief is not only missing your loved one, but it's also coming to the realization that you have to grieve the way your loved one saw you and felt about you. He says that you are also grieving the way you understood yourself when you were with them. It sounds absurd, but I had to learn how not to be the victim in a relationship that would never have any closure.

So, I thought that if I smiled enough, if I faked it then eventually it would make everything OK. I immersed myself in my job and the lives of my children and extended family, and I was determined that it was going to be fixed. Well, it was not OK. It took some time, but eventually I crashed and burned.

Emotional Self

Social Science Researcher, Dr. Brené Brown who has spent her life studying shame and vulnerability, explains that our bodies record our emotions, keeps score, and always wins. So, when you actually try to bury your emotions, instead of facing them and dealing with them, it can lead to all sorts of colorful complications. This is the reason people who have experienced a life-threatening event get diagnosed with Post Traumatic Stress Disorder (PTSD).

The inability or avoidance of dealing with the messy work can lead to all sorts of depression, anxiety, drastic weight gain or loss, over and under eating, and lack of sleep—just to name a few complications. Inevitably, right on cue that is when it all began. I cannot pinpoint the day I met Depression. It came in seemingly uninvited and helped itself to my feelings, my hair, my weight, and my smile.

I often wonder what my life would be like if I had not met Depression at that particular time in my life. Depression gets around, so you may have made its acquaintance. It is always lurking and always looking for a way in. Depression does not care what has or has not happened in your life. It does not care if you are grieving the loss of a loved one or a job. It could care less about where you work or if you even work at all. Depression wants to be your bestie. Your BFF (best friend forever). It wants to be there until the end. It wants to be your end. It is misery and you are company.

Depression is to life what weeds are to a healthy garden. I absolutely love gardening. As a gardener, I have planted many seeds. Some plants flourish right where I plant them, and others need special care. I often have to make the decision to move a plant to a different location so that I can cater to its unique needs. Often times, especially in my neck of the woods, the weather is unpredictable. This unpredictable weather is just like the unfortunate circumstances that enter our lives when we least expect it.

But, there will always be weeds. Weeds are simply plants that are in the wrong place. They are undesirable to gardeners because they can take over the garden and smother the cultivated plants by robbing them of sunlight and minerals in the soil. Weeds show up despite our best actions sometimes. A master gardener is vigilant in pulling those weeds and often times laying down products and using essential tools that will prevent the weeds from showing up in the first place.

Despite your unique set of circumstances, you are the master gardener of your life. You are not a plant therefore you can move away from the weeds that seek to choke the life out of you. If your situation is one where you are unable to move, then you can pull the weeds as they appear. Weeds and weather are going to happen to a garden no matter what.

When Dwayne passed away, my doctor and I came up with a treatment plan to treat Depression with antidepressants. Antidepressants work by balancing chemicals in your brain called neurotransmitters that affect mood and emotions. These depression medicines can help improve your mood, help you sleep better, and increase your appetite and concentration.

At first, the pills helped me to get through my days without feeling like I had a dark cloud raining down on me. However, no amount of antidepressants can stop bad weather. Weather happens, right? There are a few other ways I preserve my sanity when Depression stops by unannounced that in no way should be perceived as medical advice, but merely things that work for me with and without the use of an antidepressant.

Presently in my life, I chose to treat Depression like an acquaintance that I keep at arm's length. You know, there are friends in our lives who no matter how long we have been apart, when we see them it's like time has not passed and we can pick back up where we left off. I'm not trying to hug Depression. We will not be having coffee or watching chick flicks together. Depression is an arm's length acquaintance that I see every once in a while. I might even wave when I see it coming from across the room, but I keep IT there.

I now know to quickly retreat into a good book or deep breathing exercise that I have learned in meditation. Sometimes, more often than not, I cry.

Crying is not a sign of weakness as I had previously thought. I came to realize that crying is the body's way of cleansing. I used to cry in the shower so my kids would not see or hear me crying. I did not want them to see me being what I thought would be considered weak. I gorged myself on the lie that by not crying in front of them, I was showing them how to be strong.

What I didn't know was that it would have been appropriate to let them see me in pain. I was trying to keep everything normal, but pain is normal. Pain means you are still in the game because you still have the ability to feel. Pain means that there is a wound somewhere that is capable of going through the healing process.

Physical Self

My nutritionist says that from birth until death, the body is in always in a constant state of repair. So, when we are in pain, it is our body's way of telling us it is fixing something. Physical pain means that this wound would eventually start to heal and form a scab that would fall off and reveal the new and improved skin underneath.

Nevertheless, I wanted to keep everyone smiling. In my grieving mind, I thought that if we were all smiling then that meant that no one was hurting. I thought it meant that we were better and ready for the world again. In actuality, you cannot get away from grief any more than plants can get away from the weather. You have to, as Timothy Shriver says, face grief and transform it. You have to prepare for the weather by changing your perception of how to deal with it. What tools will you use to preserve yourself?

A vital change that happens when the usual way of thinking about or doing something is replaced by a new and different way is called a paradigm shift. A paradigm is a fundamental belief system or a way of doing something. Stephen R. Covey in his best-selling book, The 7 Habits of Highly Effective People[6], explains that the most important part of shifting a paradigm or a way of thinking is to simply give yourself a new role. He acknowledges that to make small changes one has to pay particular attention to their attitudes and behaviors. He goes on to say in order to make significant and powerful life altering changes, you have to change your paradigm or your way of thinking.

Our spiritual and emotional self has a memory just like our physical bodies. I made small changes to my physical appearance like getting new haircuts or buying new outfits. I read and created affirmations for myself to bring about healthy changes in my behavior and attitude. It was only when I chose to shift my way of thinking about depression that I made lasting progress in my life.

In 1990, Grammy Award winning singer Gloria Estefan broke her back in an accident that involved a semi-truck and her tour bus. She recollects that part of the reason she was able to recover from such a devastating injury was because she had previously been committed to weight training. Her physical self was so strong that it remembered how to get back to its original state, and her doctors reported that she was able to heal much quicker because of her training before the accident.

Diet and nutrition play an important role in keeping your physical self healthy. My nutritionist explained to me that the human body has fat cells that have a memory. This is one of the reasons it is so easy for our bodies to gain weight after a diet. Our bodies actually remember being a certain size so as soon as we return to that comfortable unhealthy way of eating, we not only gain the weight back, but we put on extra pounds as well.

Similarly, I have heard people say that they are predisposed to certain diseases such as heart attacks, strokes, and diabetes to name a few—all due to their family history. How revolutionary it would be to shift your paradigm to a healthier lifestyle. More often than not, we fall victim to the same diseases of our forefathers because we inherit the same unhealthy lifestyle they had. I envision a world where future generations would not succumb to those familial diseases.

I also joined a national non-profit organization called Girltrek. Girltrek's mission is to transform the lives of women of color by encouraging women to walk at least 30 minutes per day, preferably in the sunlight. I came to realize that exercise naturally produces the same feel good endorphins in your brain that antidepressants synthetically produce. The reason we exercise outside is because studies show that twenty minutes of exposure to sunlight have been proven to help with feelings of melancholy. A lack of sunlight can actually lead to a form of clinical depression. The less sunlight we see in the winter months, the more likely we are to develop Seasonal Affective Disorder (SAD). Symptoms of SAD can be extreme: mood swings, anxiety, sleep problems, or even suicidal thoughts. The transformation in my thinking took place when I truly began to view

Girltrek as more than just an exercise program, but a lifestyle change.

Spiritual Self

Our spiritual selves have a memory as well. My mother often says that we should make it a point to fully embrace the spiritual nature of any and all that we experience throughout life. All Christian denominations speak of generational curses and spiritual warfare. In the Old Testament, the American Standard Version (ASV) of the Bible states in Exodus 34:7 that God "visits the iniquity of the fathers upon the children and the children's children to the third and fourth generation."

It can be unsettling to think that the skeletons in my family's closet can come back to haunt myself, my children, and my children's children. However, in the same manner that we do not have to attribute certain "hereditary" diseases to bad genes, we do not have to be held accountable for the sins of our forefathers.

As Christians, it is a fundamental belief that one merely has to call upon the name of the Lord (Roman 10:13) to be saved. Just as with the emotional and physical areas of our lives, spiritually there is a change of mindset from the readings in the Old Testament which lays down the foundation to the New Testament. The whole Bible is the inspired Word of God and, like our lives, it is progressive. Similar to the first part of our lives, there was a lot to be learned in the Old Testament. The first part of Bible contained stories and laws that had to be lived in order to lay foundation for the stories of the New Testament to be told. This is evident in 2 Corinthians 5:17 which the Apostle Paul proclaims, "Therefore, if anyone is in Christ, the new creation has come: The old has gone, the new is here!"

Our spiritual, emotional, and physical selves have a memory. I now know that to change or fix anything about myself I had to drastically alter and nurture my beliefs about spirituality, my mental health, and my physical abilities. So, if my emotional self has a memory, and I went through some sort of trauma, it is crucial that I find a way to bring about a paradigm shift in my emotional self. I can pull those weeds by seeking the help of a person that is a coach or a specialist in that field. What I know for sure is that doing nothing about it can lead to catastrophic events that hinder me from living my best life and fulfilling my purpose.

⫸ ⫸ ⫸

It is absolutely acceptable to be, as I am, a magnificent work in progress. I have faith and I trust in God as He guides me to pull weeds as I see them by distancing myself from the things that make them appear in the first place. I find someone that can help like a close friend with positive values, a therapist, an inspirational family member, or a life coach. It is not okay to naively think that you can fix traumatic experiences on your own. I have found a great deal of solace in meditation as well.

When a child has difficulty with schoolwork a parent may tutor that child or find a tutor to help. As mothers, when our children are sick we immediately start finding ways to ease their discomfort but often neglect to find ways to help ourselves. Likewise, when I taught elementary school, if I witnessed a student having a difficult time I often found another student to pair the student up with that I knew would cause a shift in their mood in a positive and lasting way. To bring about a fundamental change in my life, I stopped ignoring the pain and I embraced it as an assurance that the healing had begun. This was not a realization I came to overnight. It was a truth that materialized over time once I changed the way I thought about grief and depression. It was a gradual shift that started with my behaviors and attitudes and manifested into a life altering paradigm shift.

In essence, I stopped trying to fix the things that I could not control. I cannot, despite my best efforts, control the weather but I can prepare for the weather by dressing appropriately. Even if I did not know a storm was brewing and I wake up to discover the sky is falling, I would not go out in the elements unprepared. I would work to find a solution for the problem because, like the weather, there are things that happen in life that cannot be avoided. Just as faith without works is dead (James 2:20), or a body builder must be consistent to work on his/her physique, we must find new and satisfying ways to grow and learn.

Chapter Six

Coping with Grief

by Amber N. Warner

> *To honor your grief is not self-destructive or harmful, it is courageous and life-giving.*
>
> Alan D. Wolfelt, Ph.D.

Into every life some rain will fall. I have experienced my fair share of rain and there are things I have learned about life, pain and loss. These experiences could have left anyone living a broken and miserable life. Unfortunately, they happen to all of us, and when it happened to me, I wasn't expecting it.

As a married woman, healthcare professional, and sorority girl with lots of caring friends, I still felt alone. While I don't know your present situation, I do know you are not alone. And maybe there might be one thing I have learned that helps you take that next step forward in your healing process. As a matter of fact, in full disclosure, I'm writing this just as much for you as I am for myself, for I'm still healing. I have had to commit myself to healing every day in order to bring my best self to the present moment. Some days the effort is easier than others, yet it is still a daily commitment of self-awareness.

We are more alike than we know. It's the common ground where healing and acceptance grow. When we put our guard down and share authentically, change and understanding can meet. So, if you can relate to losing someone you love suddenly, losing someone you love slowly, and having to let go of your idea of how you thought your life was supposed to be, then there is something for you in what I have to share.

>⢀⢀ >⢀⢀ >⢀⢀

While I have a very large extended family, my immediate family is very small. Here we may be different. Maybe your family is large with lots of beautiful siblings, in-laws and aunts or uncles, that difference doesn't matter. The difference is irrelevant because the pain of loss doesn't differentiate based on family size.

However, it is important to note that I am my mother's only biological child. Just saying that sounds lonely. On my mother's side, I have an aunt, who had no children, and my grandmother. On my biological father's side, I have a brother 10 years younger than me, an uncle with two children, the eldest being 15 years younger than me, and my grandparents.

My first loss was that there were no huge family reunions for us when I was growing up! And seriously

I always wished for this. Perhaps it was the love from my extended family that taught me how to love my immediate family so much and long for these types of family gatherings. I have always desired and wanted my family to ALL be together.

I was 10 years old when my paternal grandfather died of a massive heart attack. He wasn't more than 53 years old. That was painful, hard to comprehend and so permanent. And somehow, secretly, I thought it was my fault. Not until after studying grief and loss did I learn that it is common for children to blame themselves for death, divorce or other family issues.

That's what I did though. While I loved my grandfather, he had done some things that caused me to be angry with him for his inappropriate behavior. When he died, I was sure I had killed him because I didn't want to kiss him goodbye the last time I saw him. I was convinced my anger was wrong and I was responsible for his death.

About 10 years later, I found out my father had a terminal illness. Now, I wasn't raised by my father after the age of 2. We didn't even live in the same state or on the same coast for most of my childhood. That was a huge loss for me too, and somehow, I always held a special place in my heart for my father. I guarded that part of my heart and wouldn't let anyone in, not my mom, step father, heck not even myself.

I remember my uncle telling me that my dad was really sick. I wasn't told what the illness was, but my uncle who was more consistently like a father to me, was willing to arrange a visit for me to have a heart-to-heart conversation with my dad before he passed away. Now in my early 20's, I declined the offer. You see, when my father and I would talk, I was the one always doing the calling. I was tired of being the adult in the relationship. I didn't feel it was necessary for me to have some last conversation with him on his death bed. My uncle, being concerned but wanting to respect my decision at the time, left the offer open for me; and whenever, if ever, I wanted to make that trip, he was willing to help me get there.

I was in graduate school and found a church home that valued teaching from the Bible. I started attending church regularly. I began to study and learn the Bible for myself and that was the difference from all the other times I had been in church. To say that understanding the Bible for myself has been a blessing for me is true yet an understatement. For me, the Bible was essential in my transformation and change of heart. It taught me about forgiveness and, in order to have all of the blessings from Father God, I needed to deal with my earthly father.

I started out on a journey of self-discovery, healing and getting questions answered by my earthly father to reconcile loss, grief, hurt and abandonment through the art of forgiveness. In the midst of this, I was becoming closer with my biological father. Through my biological father's illness, our relationships were being reconciled. My uncle and father were getting closer. My paternal grandmother was visiting the West coast more often. We were even planning a family reunion. As a matter of fact, everyone was in San Diego, California just waiting on me to finish graduate school that summer, then we would all be together.

I recall my uncle even teasing me that he was just talking to my dad about surprising me for my June graduation. They thought it would be fun and knew I'd be overjoyed. Oh my goodness, I was just thrilled that the idea and conversation had even come up. But... I got that call, one week before graduation... my uncle, my dad's older brother, the man who was like a father to me, 29 days after his 51st birthday died of a massive heart attack.

I have had a lot of people in my life die suddenly. My grandfather was the first person that I remember passing away. As a 10-year-old, I didn't quite realize how young he was, but when I was 46, I really started to put things in perspective and it hit me hard to know that I am not that far from that age.

>⛧ >⛧ >⛧

I graduated as a social worker and got married. It was a happy time for me. My biological dad and his mother came to my wedding. I had my whole life ahead of me. I ended up losing my dad within the first year of my marriage and a few months later, I lost his mother, my grandmother. I was working in the public school setting. I hadn't begun my grief training at the time. What I was certain of was that I didn't want anybody else to leave my life suddenly. The sense of loss was overwhelming. The grieving process of sudden death to health conditions is similar to grieving the loss of someone to suicide.

In 2003, my maternal grandmother was diagnosed with age-related dementia. I prayed so hard for her, "Please God, you can't take her away from me. I won't be able to handle that. I've handled all of this. I just can't deal with losing her too." By God's grace, He spared her a sudden death, I had her for 10 more years before she passed away; although that felt like a life time, I really began to look at my work as a clinical social worker, and trying to get started in understanding grief and helping others to cope with grief as well.

My desire to help others in this area springs out of my experiencing so much loss in a concentrated amount of time. My journey helps me better understand grief for myself, and caused me to become more aware of how others cope with their grief. One of the great influences in helping me better cope with my grief is the work of Dr. Alan Wolfelt. I was introduced to his work when I attended a grief group.

In our culture and society, we do not deal well with grief. We have all heard the following statements:

"Death is part of the process, so we live, and we die."

"Life goes on."

"You cry, and you move on and you get over it."

"The Bible tells us to focus on the living and not the dead."

I believe that those kinds of statements and others really do not help people in the grieving process. It has the opposite effect. It creates an environment in which people are shamed for feeling certain emotions. People decide that you shouldn't be feeling a certain way and then you don't have anyone that you can talk to about your grief. People, often times, feel isolated and then are at a loss as to how to deal with their grief. I've learned that talking about your experience helps and there should be no shame in experiencing and expressing grief. How a person deals with grief should not be dictated by someone else's timeline. Those affected by grief should take the time they need to process and deal with their grief regardless of what others think or anyone else's subjective timeline.

Another lesson for me and one that is often overlooked is that we grieve a lot of different types of losses. We certainly grieve death; we grieve illness, change in our abilities or those of our loved ones; we grieve lost opportunities including employment; we grieve estranged relationships; we grieve when we experience separation from something we value; we grieve the loss of our pets and so much more. When we don't acknowledge our losses and give ourselves permission to grieve and mourn, we can create additional stressors and hardships for ourselves.

Grief can be accompanied by a variety of physical symptoms. Whatsyourgrief.com and GriefWatch.com both state that physical symptoms are normal during the grieving process and may consist of fatigue, aches and pains, tightness in the chest, shortness of breath, headaches, forgetfulness, inability to focus, appetite changes, digestive issues, and getting sick more often. That's what happened to me. I initially minimized the losses I had experienced, trying to keep it all inside and to myself, hoping no one could tell of my hurt and suffering.

One night I knew the tingling in my arms was too much, coupled with the pressure I felt in my chest, I even had shortness of breath, I felt as if I was losing it, scared that maybe I was having a heart attack or even worse would have one in my sleep. While I rationalized I was having a panic attack and I could just "process" my way through this, my anxiety grew bigger at the thought of what if it was a heart attack, and I died in my sleep?

I tried to reason through my symptoms and keep calm. Just breathe through it, I thought. It wasn't working and my breath got shorter, I couldn't ignore these symptoms because heart disease runs in my family. And I had never in my life had that type of heaviness in my chest, nor tingling in my arms. The more I tried to quietly breathe, the louder I felt my head pounding the question that those symptoms may be that of a heart attack. I had to say something to my husband that night because really, the numbness in my arms had already been there for the past few days and wasn't going away.

Grief can impact your physical health if you do not attend to it. Our brain does not distinguish between emotional pain caused by grief or the physical pain caused by stubbing one's toe. Whether you experience physical or emotional pain, your brain is sent the same signal and the body is going to have similar responses. I read an article that stated, "When people feel emotional pain, the same areas of the brain get activated as when people feel physical pain: the anterior insula and the anterior cingulate cortex."[7] The good news is that there are ways that you can process and deal with your grief that are healthy and can propel you into living a richer life—and that's what I want people to know.

⤖ ⤖ ⤖

My grandmother's death hit me very hard. She was 83 years old. I'm blessed to have had her in my life. She died in my Aunt's arms from the natural progression of Alzheimer's Disease. It wasn't like I was suffering from the untimely death of a child, or the loss of a life-long partner. And yet, my grief almost knocked me upside down. I was in a lot of pain. If I could feel so devastated by my grandmother's death, a woman who lived a long life, how do others deal with their losses?

>‖> >‖> >‖>

These are topics we tend not to discuss. I have learned to check in with myself. I am naturally an emotional person. When I cry, I know that my tears have a purpose and are not always tears of sadness. Therefore, I take time to understand why I'm crying and sometimes it is because I am sad, but sometimes it's just that I'm grateful. I am grateful for the time I had with my grandmother. But, it took me a while to get there during my first year of mourning. One of the most important things that I've learned is that it's okay for me to embrace the pain when I feel it, since it comes from a space of much love.

Three months after my grandmother died, I lost my aunt, my grandmother's youngest child. My aunt was eight years older than me. My grief was no longer so-called "normal grief", it was now "complicated grief". I read about that in a book by Dr. Alan D. Wolfelt.

Dr. Wolfelt describes six needs of mourning: 1) Acknowledge the reality of the death, by gently confronting that someone you care about will never physically come back. 2) Embrace the pain of the loss, resist avoiding, denying, and repressing instead confront and reconcile to it. 3) Remember the person who died, through precious memories and objects that link you to your loved one, this allows you to pursue this relationship. 4) Develop a new self-identity, when someone with whom you have a relationship dies, the way you see yourself naturally changes. 5) Search for meaning, naturally question the meaning and purpose of life, perhaps exploring religious and spiritual values. And finally, 6) Receive ongoing support, drawing on the experience and encouragement of friends, fellow mourners or professional counselors is not a weakness, but a healthy human need.[8]

I was particularly touched by #2, embrace the pain. I realized that it was okay for me to feel hurt, sad, and an overwhelming sense of loss. I did not have to rush through it, hurry up and get over it, nor do I ever have to forget it.

In April 2013, a few days before my aunt's memorial service, I was watching the backstory of Blake Shelton, a country music artist and musical coach on the hit NBC TV show 'The Voice'. I recall, Blake's father, Richard Shelton being interviewed when he spoke of the sudden death of his son, Blake's older brother. Richard Shelton said, "Losing a child, it's something that you don't ever get over. It's something that you have to learn to live with."

In that moment, my pain connected with his and his words freed and healed me. Instead of trying to push my pain away, he gave me permission to learn from it forever. That's why I wanted to participate in this anthology project, to be able to share and be there for someone else that may be feeling or experienced something similar. To be able to encourage others to live their abundant life, too, despite the pain.

>⊪ >⊪ >⊪

One of the techniques I use personally and in my clinical practice with others experiencing grief is called dosing. Marty Tousley, an experienced grief counselor, said, "You might think about actually setting aside some time just for yourself each day – I call it your crying time – when you allow yourself to give in completely to your grief and feel whatever you need to feel, including feeling sorry for yourself. Others have referred to this as 'dosing,' and for many mourners, it can be a very effective tool as it gives you some sense of control over your grief – or at least when and how you choose to immerse yourself in your feelings of loss — and a way to contain it, too. This way, you can pick the time of day and you can decide how long it will last."[9]

In other words, grief dosing gives us permission to feel grief, but at the same time, we get to set it aside, take a break and walk away from it, so it does not consume us. You can dose your grief just like a prescription. You know you can control it. You can decide, okay, so on this day, at this time, I'm going to journal about it. You could choose to do whatever it takes to work through your grief or to honor your loved one, but then you must give yourself permission to walk away from the pain, so the pain does not become debilitating.

>>> >>> >>>

It is crucially important that you pay attention to your health. When I had the chest pain, tingling sensations, and shortness of breath, I was very concerned particularly due to my family medical history of heart disease. Although, I was pretty certain my symptoms were psychological, I was encouraged to have an electrocardiogram (EKG) from my healthcare provider. Some of us might be more vulnerable to heart disease than others and we owe it ourselves to take our health seriously and follow the recommendations of medical experts. To my dismay, my EKG was not normal and further testing was required. I was diagnosed with broken heart syndrome. My ejection fraction temporary had been functioning below the ideal rate of 60. I underwent some treatment and it went back to normal.

The Mayo Clinic, Patient Care and Health Information describes Broken Heart syndrome as "a temporary heart condition that's often brought on by stressful situations, such as the death of a loved one. The condition can also be triggered by a serious physical illness or surgery. People with broken heart syndrome may have sudden chest pain or think they're having a heart attack."[10] Who knew there was such a thing and it is not just a euphemism?

My journey to understand my grief and to help others with their grief had led me to learn from many sources. I gleaned information from counselors everywhere, hospice providers, including what I call my TV counselors or meaningful moments. I was watching a documentary on Nelson Mandela and he shared that he buried his parents right on the property which he stood, and he felt like a piece of himself was buried with them.

Hearing other people talk about their grief even on TV was insightful for me because it helped me understand and give words to the emotion I was feeling. A piece of me was gone with the passing of my grandmother and aunt, and as much as I wished the world would stop so I could catch up and adjust, I needed to learn that being uncertain and not in control was okay. I needed to allow myself to mourn and yield to time to discover how their passing would change me.

>⧓ >⧓ >⧓

I believe that coming from a small family intensified my anxiety the night of my panic attack that lead to my medical work up and being diagnosed with Broken Heart Syndrome. I recall speaking to my mother that night and she said, "It's just you and me left." We were both in shock by the passing of my aunt. In that moment I was engulfed by grief.

Loss has a way of putting things in perspective. If we are fortunate enough to have children, when we look at our children, we see our future. When we look at our grandparents and elders, we celebrate our past. When I was doing my grief work, I realized my past was slowly fading with family members passing away. And unfortunately, so was my future since I did not have biological children. While I've accepted not having biological children, I am learning that I still have grief work to do in this area.

>⧓ >⧓ >⧓

Not too long ago, I went on a medical mission to Uganda and the focus was on women's maternal health. I discovered the paramount importance motherhood is to the Ugandan women. I connected with the women we served in a special way, and I could see that they were very dedicated to have children. Many had suffered miscarriages or even had stillborn births.

As I was interviewing the women about their healthcare experience and losses, I could feel their sadness. I spoke with a 27-year-old woman who had experienced a stillbirth the day before. In asking how was she doing she replied, "I'm feeling some type of way, but I am going to be okay." Interestingly enough, I felt I knew the place where she was coming from and from her verbal expression, she gave voice to the grief that was inside me at times.

Sometimes, we withdraw into our grief. We may close out our spouse, friends, siblings, parents and loved ones. Grief can be an isolating experience and when we isolate ourselves, it tears at the seams of our relationships. As those relationships become more fragile or crumble, we experience even more pain, more grief. It can be a vicious and never-ending cycle if we don't learn how to grieve in a way that lends to our health, deeper connections and a fulfilling life.

>⧽ >⧽ >⧽

So, how did I deal with my grief? I accepted the reality that my loved ones had transitioned and I could continue my relationship with them through my memories and meaningful objects. As I felt the pain from loss and I talked about that while actively listening to others that are grieving, I actively embraced the positive in my life personally and professionally.

For example, although I do not have biological children, I call myself a mother to many. I have a habit of spiritually mentoring/adopting "other peoples' children". I am a big sister, auntie, mentor or mother figure. Contributing to our village, completes me and helps me to heal and share resources. I try to serve and lighten the load of others. I am grateful to be where I am in life to be able to bless and help someone else. Having an attitude of gratitude helps me maintain a healthy grief balance, being thankful and appreciative for the time and influence I had with my family has been a gift.

I had to begin to embrace the positives, while I have listed many above, they were not always easy to uncover, although they were always there. We must always look for the positives, although they don't scream at us like the negatives do! Right?

If you have read this chapter and it is stirring up unresolved feelings for you, may I suggest that you review The Six Needs of Mourning, identify any of the needs you have made progress, and celebrate that accomplishment. Are any of the needs challenging for you? If so, how and why, and decide what you want to do about that.

Remember to practice dosing with your grief, set aside a specific amount of time and place for you to explore and express your emotions and pain. Be gentle with yourself. Grieving is normal and part of the human experience. It is universal yet unique. Mourning can take days, months and years.

Most importantly connect with someone you trust and that is an active listener. Do not be afraid to seek professional help at any time. If you are consumed with grief and it is hindering your productivity at work, home, self-care and/or socially, and you are unsure of how to contact for assistance, call the Grief Recovery Helpline 1-800-445-4808. Phone numbers can change without notice, in that case, please call your local information number, or google the crisis line in your area.

Thank you for allowing me to share my experience. I encourage you to find something first that feels safe so that you can begin your journey of self-discovery. I hope you uncover that you are not alone. Remember loss is not something we have to get over, it's something we must learn to live with. You can live your abundant life even in the midst of loss.

Chapter Seven

Taking Back My Power

by Laura L. Johnson

> *Life is 10% what happens to you and 90% how you react to it.*
>
> *Charles R. Swindoll*

People in every area of life are struggling. Often, events beyond our control or understanding play a part to make us feel like we are in a prison from our past. We feel alone in our pain, ashamed to tell how we have been hurt or possibly hurt others. Depression sets in, sometimes we lash out at the ones we love the most, transferring our pain to another.

God says, "…I will never leave thee, nor forsake thee." [Hebrews 13:5 KJV]

You are NOT alone. The path your life has taken is a direct result of the influences in your life, your surroundings, and how you perceive and process your environment.

I've been asked how I feel "entitled" to speak about "hard" subjects such as sexual molestation, rape, addiction, abortion, overeating, shame, domestic violence, and suicide—just to name a few.

My answer? "I'm an overcomer from the school of hard knocks. I wasn't prepared for where my life had taken me, I learned each day how to make the best of situations and do my best to only speak on subjects I personally have dealt with, knowing God is by my side."

⫸ ⫸ ⫸

I spent many years in denial that I was in any pain, that I had anything to hide from the world. I was in denial that I ever hurt anyone. That denial cost me a heavy price. By keeping "secrets" from myself, I allowed the "ripple effects" of my pain to spill over into the lives of others.

I found a lot of ways to cope with my pain. I blocked many experiences from my memory, stuffed down my emotions and refused to feel. I used food to comfort myself; and used drugs, alcohol, anger, sex and lies to self-medicate. I wallowed in self-pity, used the dangerous game of "excuse and accuse". I became a professional victim.

Today, I openly own up to my pain and take responsibility for my life; accepting that many things were completely out of my control. Only then have I began to heal, by the grace of God.

I pray that the incidents in my life and the revelation I have received will break down barriers in your life and the lives of others. My prayers are for restoration in marriages, relationships with parents, siblings, and children. May the "secret" chains of your bondage be broken, fall away, and your mind and heart be set free from your past! Let my story release you from your sinful hurts, habits, and hang-ups. Let your addictions be a part of the past and let the glorious light of God shine into your heart!

>₪⊳ >₪⊳ >₪⊳

Be strong and courageous. Do not be afraid or terrified because of them, for the LORD your God goes with you; He will never leave you nor forsake you. [Deuteronomy 31:6 NIV]

My story begins in a small rural town of Milton, Florida to parents nearly a decade apart in age. My dad was 27 years old when I was born. My mother had just turned 16. She grew up and matured as my sisters and I grew. A good-hearted, humble and meek woman with a smoldering, underlying rage trying to cope with her own demons of sexual molestation and brutality.

My parents used corporal punishment and I was taught manners, respect and good morals at their hands. I knew they loved me and wanted only the best for me. I saw their day-to-day struggle with life and empathized with them from a young age. Switches (real thin tree stems/branches that were bendable) and leather belts were a normal form of punishment for us.

As a 4-year-old, I was brutally sodomized by my maternal grandfather. I remember the confusion as I was commanded to undress and bend over the old metal footboard of my childhood bed. The ugly greasy stain on my mothers' hand bleached hardwood floors will forever remain in my heart and mind as I tried to block out the searing pain and scream through the madness where my face was being pushed into the mattress.

I tried to fight each time I was left alone with him but, he was 6'4" and 280 pounds of ugly big beefy beast with work-roughened hands and alcohol breath. I didn't stand a chance. At age eight, I threatened him with calling the police as I saw the signs he was "grooming" my sisters for the same horror. This nightmare in the flesh left me traumatized each time he raped me. I became afraid of older men, I lashed out in anger, I hid under houses, in trees, and in the unlocked car and shed that belonged to our neighbor.

I began to eat as a way to comfort myself. Trying to hide the vulnerable child in an ugly unwanted body— it didn't work. This is a self-medicating tactic I still use 54 years later. I tried to hide the abused child with a mask of "I'm fine."

That same attitude and fear caused me to keep quiet when I was raped by a childhood friend at the age of 13. Matter of fact, I can recall moments where I can clearly remember my abusers and attempted abusers, many friends of the family and relatives, who had "touchy-feely" hands and lascivious looks. A look I now identify as a ravenous wolf or rabid dog. Thirsty. Evil. Painful. Cruel.

⫸ ⫸ ⫸

I have vague memories of my paternal grandparents taking me to church. We stayed in their home until they passed away. May God bless the praying persons' soul a thousand times over. God hears all things.

I must have been "dedicated" to God around that time as He carried me through so many difficult and harsh realities in the months and years to come. Without Him, I know I would have never made it.

≫⊪ ≫⊪ ≫⊪

Do not fear, for I am with you; do not anxiously look about you, for I am your God. I will strengthen you, surely I will help you, surely I will uphold you with My righteous right hand. [Isaiah 41:10 NIV]

At the age of 17, I met my first boyfriend—he loved loving me and we explored each other gently with "puppy love", until we were forced apart when his parents moved hundreds of miles away. I was sexually addicted. I thought I had finally found total love and acceptance, only to be deceived.

I joined the United States Army's delayed enlistment program the first semester of my junior year of high school, which meant there was a two-year wait while I finished high school. While in high school, I was in the Navy Junior Reserve Officers Training Corps (NJROTC). I joined the rifle team and went on to letter in Rifle expertise (a letter to place on my 'brag jacket'), and ladies drill team of both armed and unarmed guard. I stayed busy and kept a low profile. Yet, still, I searched relentlessly for love and affection, becoming promiscuous in my senior year.

Before graduation, I moved out of my parents' home, happy not to hear the daily arguments and accusations of two people trying to survive a life they were never prepared for. But the Army presented a whole new kind of adventure after graduation, there was anything you could desire, except morals.

During my first year in the Army, I matured a lot but not enough! I started drinking after work, playing cards and having random sex... searching for a "love of my own". I had no experience drinking hard liquor except for the watered down drinks my molesting grandfather used to force me to drink after the assaults to "make me feel better".

As a result, I was alcohol poisoned. I drank a lot fast and blacked out! The next thing I remember was looking up to see emergency room lights above me and an oxygen mask on my face. I overheard the emergency room doctor saying, "Another thirty minutes and we'd have another soldier gone."

I received a disciplinary action that cost me three month's pay, admitted to rehab, and barred me from carrying a weapon. While in rehab, I found out that I was pregnant. Upon completion of the intense daily group meeting and psychoanalysis, I returned to my duty station in New York. Waiting for me upon my return were four upper level sergeants and the lieutenant I previously had an altercation with; and their mission was solely to intimidate me into getting an abortion. They used fear, guilt and shame by pointing out that I came from a small hometown, and returning with an illegitimate baby would be a great burden to my parents. Their scare tactics worked and I agreed to have an abortion.

That experience left me traumatized. I remember waking up at night listening—not realizing that I was listening for my baby boy that I aborted. I would literally go looking for him around the house and everywhere else I went. That went on for weeks, and even now, some 38 years later, I still look for him occasionally.

I heard babies cry... I felt alone, something was missing. Tears in the night. Sorrow. Shame. Trauma. The guilt haunted me day in and day out. Finally, I submitted a request to transfer to another post. I was sent to Frankfurt, Germany. Oh, how I thought I was escaping, only to finally figure out that location wasn't the cause of my problems. My traumatized mindset followed me.

>⧉ >⧉ >⧉

I was insane. Let me give you a definition here: Insanity is doing the same thing over and over and expecting different results. Within 90 days, I was back to drinking and having casual sex. I ended up pregnant again—this time by a married man. Being selfish enough not to want to sacrifice my new lifestyle of drinking, marijuana, occasional 8-ball of cocaine and hard liquor black outs to end, I made the decision to have another abortion.

When I arrived at the clinic in Holland, I had no idea what to expect. The nurse there told me if I continue getting pregnant, I should learn how to perform at home procedures to abort a child. The advice I got from her would later be put to use in a manner that would cause much pain and grief.

Pausing to reflect here, I repeatedly put myself through this physical, mental and emotional abuse. I hurt. I had hardened my heart like Pharoah in the Bible. I had mental and emotional scars in my mind and branded on my heart from the foolishness of addictions. Addictions to sex, men, alcohol, drugs, and the 'hunt and conquest' drama.

And Then There Was Marriage

After returning home from the Army, I married a man from my hometown. He was a fine specimen of a man, 5'7" and muscular, clean-cut, neatly trimmed mustache and goatee, and had a teasingly wicked smile that melted my heart from day one. We were both from near poverty-level homes. He came from a strict family with a lot of hardships. We had no business together. Now I can see that, but back then we were both blinded—me by the desire for love and commitment, and him for the desire to have a steady source of income and children.

Our first daughter and oldest child, Delicia, was born on September 22, 1985. My second daughter, Tawanna, was born 21 months later on May 19, 1987. My husband was always looking for ways to steal my joy. I had no idea the lengths I'd go to stay with him because I was 'old school'—he was the father of my children, I thought he would change, and I thought I had nowhere to go. After all, we were married!

Our life on the outside was perfect. He stopped working. I worked, paid off our car, kept the bills at bay, provided a home for us. He drank, partied and often moved in with other women for 3-6 months at a time. I was a fool for the man and took his harsh abuse, trying desperately to hang on to the idea of *Prince Charming*.

>⫸ >⫸ >⫸

I must pause and tell you of one of my biggest shames that haunts me until this very day. When my oldest daughter was four months old, I got pregnant— I didn't know how far and I didn't care—I was scared. I was working, paying bills, taking verbal and physical abuse at the hands of my husband and could not possibly see having a second child in that environment. I performed the procedure the nurse in Holland had so callously taught me.

Into the 2nd week after the self-inflicted abortion, the pains began. I was at home alone with my four month old daughter, who slept through it all. I experienced full birth pains, no medication, huge clots, back spasms, total and complete discomfort.

Finally, after about 6 hours, the whole placenta, baby and all was born. The baby I thought I aborted two weeks prior. I freaked out! I took the placenta (baby still inside) to the hospital. I had to have a Dilation and Curettage (D&C). I was so embarrassed, ashamed and hurt. A deep depression settled on me like a cloak, I distinctly remember a feeling as if the sun had gone behind a cloud, and as if my shoulders were now weighed down by the weight and sorrows of the world. I had to survive for my daughter, Delicia, I pretended I was okay... yet waking in the night screaming, or crying—often both. A time in my life that I will never forget, and never reconcile.

>‖> >‖> >‖>

Back to my marriage: So when my husband figured out I couldn't have any more children, the real beatings began. I had been hit with glass ashtrays, belts, switches, chains, fists, a lamp, a car and numerous other objects thrown at me, often leaving deep gouges scratched into my face.

Over the course of the 10 years, I lived with him off and on. I had 3 broken eardrums, 6 broken ribs, and broken teeth. Once I was tied up, drugged and forced to have lesbian and bestial sex for the price of a small rock of cocaine for my husband. I'd lost 3 jobs because I couldn't be seen in public looking like that! I learned to apply makeup over bruises, to wear long sleeve shirts and long pants in the summer. I learned not to flinch timidly when something approached my area unexpectedly.

I felt like a complete failure as a mother; I allowed my children to see and hear those things for almost 10 years. At which point, I ran and moved away for two weeks. Upon my return, my house had been ransacked and all items of value were once again stolen and pawned to support his habits. He knew I meant business that time and stayed away. I worked. I buried myself in 14-16 hour days as a truck driver. I maintained a great job, bought a house, and a new car.

That time I was strong enough, thanks be to God alone, not to allow him back in my life. Folks, all that glitters is not gold! He was beautiful, dressed nice, talked eloquently, could sing like a bird. I wanted that man. I got that pain. Truth be told, I felt that Blues singer Betty Wright was right when she said, "No pain, No gain".

I endured the physical beatings, the emotional ups and downs, the cheating; and I gained life experience, shame, heartache. When I finally left, I was lonely and I would often second guess myself. Should I take him back? Was it really that bad? Seeing my children burst into hysterical tears upon seeing their dad was my final answer! I moved on. I endured.

>⠇⠇> >⠇⠇> >⠇⠇>

Soon I was involved with another man who would take a large chunk of my life and waste it on a dream. I met Karl in 1996, four months before my dad passed away. Karl was another fine specimen at 6'4", muscular, long soft braids—he was my kryptonite. I should have recognized the red flags of bragging, fighting, drinking to drunkenness each night, and controlling my actions through fear.

God was walking beside me softly calling my name at that time I know, but I refused to hear from Him. I had no true understanding of God, though I attempted to understand and study many religions over the years. But the question still remained: why wasn't I able to find joy and happiness?

February 8, 2004, I found myself on my hands and knees at an altar call for a wedding. I was the only one of about 100 guests on my knees—tears, mascara, and boogers running down my face. It was my time. I FINALLY heard His soft whisper to my heart! I stopped drinking that very day.

⫸ ⫸ ⫸

I've often heard that a robber has no reason to steal from a deserted house, after all what would they get? By that same token, I believe the enemy saw what God created me for and, even though I still walk without full understanding, I think the enemy was trying to make me fall from my newly found Father.

He took my mother thirty days after I was saved on March 24, 2004. I was devastated. I was alone again. I had nightmares and anxiety attacks back in 1996 when my dad succumbed to lung cancer. This time, the nightmares wouldn't let me fall asleep at night. I broke out into hives. I was grumpy. I lashed out at my children, at Karl, at everybody. I was hurt and broken, I felt like everything in my life came tumbling down.

What was it all for? Why hadn't I spent more quality time with my mother? Why did the enemy take her?

About six months later I moved to Texas, hoping for a change of scenery and a change of life. I forgot that wherever I go—there I am. My habits and problems came with me.

Karl and I parted ways after he threw a bowl of ice cream at me out of anger. All of my old triggers—fear, anger, self-preservation—stepped into the forefront of my mind! I made him leave, only to find out he had been cheating the entire time. His loss.

I walked away. I was made to be cherished, loved and protected. All I had ever known was use and abuse. At 58, I'm pretty jaded about love. I know there's someone for me I just have occasional problems believing I'll ever meet him.

I've spent the last 7 years working on myself. Working out my anger. Learning to trust. Those men were handsome, well-educated men. Looking good on the outside, but deadly on the inside.

⤜ ⤜ ⤜

Through it all, and trust me, there's so much more, I knew God was by my side this time. I allowed my understanding of God's Word to catch up with my book knowledge. The woman I am determined to be has cost me a few things. It cost me some relationships that aren't healthy or encouraging, and material things I once thought might make me happy.

Today, I speak in small churches and small outings. Public speaking is a huge part of my therapy in life. It puts me smack dab in front of a huge group with nothing to hide behind. It makes me vulnerable to the opinions of others and, at the same time, it boosts my confidence. My story has touched others who've felt the same switches, rapes, beatings, shame and fear, and scalding tears in the darkest most silent of nights.

God has restored my relationship with both of my daughters. He blessed me to have three wonderful "Grand Loves"—two handsome grandsons and a beautiful princess! For this I am grateful. I have begged their forgiveness for the things I put them through as children and young adults. I asked them to forgive me for enabling them to live as they did, and not teaching them to give 1,000 percent to everything they do. Each day, God places a hedge of protection around my family. He blesses me with their safety, shelter, food and finances being taken care of.

Now unto Him that is able to keep you from falling, and to present you faultless before the presence of His glory with exceeding joy, To the only wise God our Saviour, be glory and majesty, dominion and power, both now and ever. Amen. [Jude 24-25 KJV]

You have the power to design your life with your words. I am loved. I am worthy. I am enough. I'll walk with the grace of a queen instead of the grief of a child. I am beautiful. I am saved. I am grateful. I am blessed. I am royalty. I am an overcomer. I am a survivor. I am going to reach my potential. I Am His Princess.

I AM TAKING BACK MY POWER TO LIVE MY ABUNDANT LIFE TOO!!

Tears

Poem written by Laura Louise Johnson on
February 18, 2018

Tears come in moments of great Joy.

Tears come in moments of great sadness.

Tears come when we are all alone...

Tears come when we see someone else hurts before us.

Tears come when we least expect them.

Tears come when our sentiments are great.

Tears come to smear the inked words on the lines we
write,

Tears come in the dead of night, our sleep they fight.

Tears come when Our Happiness can't be spoken.

Tears come when Old chains are Broken.

Tears my friend, tear down our walls.

Tears express our heart when we've given our all.

Tears help us to Celebrate—often salting our Birthday
cake.

Some are just words only my eyes can make, making
us shake.

Some slide down our face as slow rivers of grief and
pain,

Some come falling like the hardest of the Rains.

Sometimes we cry because we must say goodbye...

A home, a friend—even a butterfly...

Tears are often just an expression of how we feel.

Each tear is a story that's real...

Not always a war we've fought, usually referencing an answer we've sought.

Tears dear Lord that are mine, turn into smiles showing I'm fine.

Every tear that we've cried, is caught in the Hands of God.

Returned to us purified, healing to us as they fall...

Tears my friend, tear down our walls.

Tears are often just a release.maybe we just need a squeeze...

Lord , Help me shed some tears... Please...

Wash me, Lord, Set me Free...

Chapter Eight

I Am More Than My Vagina

by Shalita Randall

> *The Lord is my light and my salvation whom shall I fear? The Lord is the strength of my life; of whom shall I be afraid?*
>
> *Psalm 27:1 (KJV)*

Dedicated to: Every young girl who was taught your PACKAGING is more important than your GIFT

I am more than my vagina. It's a bold statement but it takes a lot of girls a long time to get that revelation. God created us women with beauty and strength, multifaceted and very intelligent. Not to be exploited, abused, misused, raped, or degraded.

My first memory of sexual awareness and vagina was at the hands of my stepsister. I was about four or five years old. Raised in a poor family. I have seven biological siblings, two step sisters, and three of my cousins were raised with us. If you lost count, that's fifteen people under one roof. A roof that sometimes had no light, or running water, one where the refrigerator was filled with discarded food from dumpsters. Yes, we literally dug out the dumpsters to eat!

I remember once when the lights were cut off, one of my older sisters made tuna and crackers by the candle. She bent over too far and her hair caught fire. She rolled on the bed and used her poncho to smother the fire. In that moment it was scary, but we laugh about it today.

Vagina, when you're a young girl, four or five, you're aware that you have one but not fully comprehending what it's for. So, you can imagine that when my stepsister opened her legs and told me to lick it, I had no clue what I was doing. Though there were that many children in the home, ages ranging from fifteen to infant, sex was a taboo topic. You would think that one would educate their children, and make them realize that children before preparation could equal poverty.

>⊪ >⊪ >⊪

So, let's start from the beginning. I was born in the 80's to a mom who had her first child at the age of fourteen. I was number five, and all of us were birthed out of wedlock. None of us were raised with our biological fathers in the picture. Until this very day all I know of my father is his name and that he died from cancer. I have no idea where he's buried or if I have other siblings in the world.

Somewhere along the way my mom became involved with a wolf in sheep's clothing. He added his two daughters to the mix and together they had three more. Now add the three cousins and that's the way we became the antithesis of the Brady Bunch.

The wolf, that monster that haunts you when you're awake. They called him "Rev", yes, he was known as a preacher. A preacher is supposed to be a pillar of the community. Someone people can look up to for moral and spiritual guidance. This wolf was a predator, and his prey was the innocent virgins in our family. He would preach fire and brimstone in the pulpit. He would even speak in tongues and lay hands on people. He used the same Jesus he preached about to try and brainwash us.

We weren't allowed to date, or wear make-up. For a while when we were growing up, we weren't allowed to wear pants. Now from the outside looking in, that may seem normal. Sure, he's a shepherd of God's flock, they tend to be protective of their daughters, not a wolf. A wolf used that to be controlling. *Don't do anything that may attract someone to you. I don't want them to take you before I had my chance to pounce on you.*

In front of an audience, meaning anyone who was around at the time, he was charismatic, intelligent, book smart, and street smart. Behind closed doors, he was emotionally, mentally, and physically abusive. It made no difference your age or gender. Nor did your position in the family matter. His wrath had no boundaries.

One day my oldest sister and I stayed home from school. All I recall is the wolf with one hand around my mother's throat and the other hand punching her in the face. All the while he's literally dragging her through the house. My sister and I were terrified, all we could do was cry. Did my mother leave him? Did she take her kids and walk away? No, not by any means.

So, the vagina issue was presented with me as the culprit. I was told I was wrong, I was being bad. I needed to stop that. I was labelled as having the spirit of lesbianism. I learned that who I was didn't matter, I wasn't worth fighting for. Nobody got punished, there was no reprimand. I also learned that women were only punching bags and vagina.

You see, your parents are supposed to teach you what you need to do to live. You are then supposed to decide how you want to live. The wolf raised us to be controlled, not to be strong women. Sadly, my mom didn't know how to live. So instead, she taught me how to endure and survive. In enduring, you bottle up who you are to protect yourself from who they are. In survival, you adapt to your environment or situation. In endurance and survival, you can often develop bad habits that can sabotage your future. I developed a bad habit of not telling anyone anything bad that was going on.

I didn't tell anyone about my near rape experience in the ninth grade. I was walking to class minding my business and a guy pulled me in the restroom. In a frantic almost animal-like way, frustration tried to undress me. Thanks be to Heaven, nothing happened. He didn't get any clothes off and I wasn't physically hurt. I was mentally, and emotionally scarred. I was scared and shocked, worst of all, I knew him. So, I kept my mouth shut.

I didn't tell anyone about my near consensual sex moment. I was in the tenth grade, he too pulled me into the restroom. He tried to undress me. I said no, I was too scared. I kept thinking I might get pregnant because we had no protection. We had no business being alone in that way.

My biggest mistake was not telling anyone when this wolf, this predator decided to pounce on me. I was terrified of him, I had seen his rage and abuse before. I had been on the receiving of that rage. So that day which was a Sunday, I remember because everyone else went to church.

He had a business, if that's what you want to call it. It was a small store front, and in the corner there was a bench out of sight of any door or window. He laid me down and tore my virginity away from me. I remember being sore and going to the restroom to wipe away the blood. When everyone else came back from church, we kept living as if nothing had happened.

What I didn't understand about this exchange, was that it wouldn't be the only occurrence. I had no clue what to do, but somehow, I knew it wasn't right. Again, all he wanted was my packaging, my vagina. I developed another bad habit, promiscuity.

⤞ ⤞ ⤞

This went on for over a year or so. I recall after one exchange, the wolf put a hickey on my neck. My mother saw it on my neck and inquired about it. She specifically said, "Your daddy been messing with you, ain't he?" I said, "Yes ma'am." I guess they exchanged words about it, but in the end, she chose him over me. There was no knock out, drawn out fight to the death. She didn't call the police. The whole concept was swept under the rug. Consequently, I became very depressed and suicidal. I didn't know who to turn to. My own mother neglected to do her one major duty as a mom—and that's to protect her child.

>⊪ >⊪ >⊪

So where do I go from here? I can't stay but I have no one to turn to. So, for my own sanity, I ran away from home. I had the goal and dream to graduate college. Somewhere in me I knew I was something better than all of this. Here I was with so many bad habits and survival "skills." I was depressed, suicidal, promiscuous, no self-confidence or self-esteem, and a vagina.

Today, I am age thirty-seven and winning at life on so many levels. I am a veteran, a college graduate, mother of one, divorced, and a home owner. With many trials and tribulations in the process but always making progress.

How did I begin to begin? I had to take accountability for my entire being. I had to stop valuing myself based on someone's measurement. Accountability for mind, body, emotions, soul, spirit, and finances. I had to understand that I was worth fighting for myself. I couldn't depend on anyone else fighting for me. I declared my peace, sanity, and freedom are non-negotiable. I made two relationships sacred: me and God, me and myself. This wasn't an act of conceit or selfishness. This was an act of self-care.

No one but you can step in and say enough is enough. Only you can do that for yourself.

Spiritual Accountability

Embrace solitude and silence. Enjoy time with God and yourself. Stop letting someone else determine your value. Determine your value with your own measuring cup.

I had to get my relationship right with God. I prayed, "Lord, please forgive me for just surviving and not living. Lord, allow me to forgive those who have hurt or harmed me in any way. Lord, teach me how to live and enjoy life. Lord, deliver me from all the dark places my life has taken me. Lord, forgive me for not fighting for myself. Give me the strength, the will, and the courage to keep going. Lord, thank You for protecting me from myself and loving me when I couldn't do it for myself. Lord, teach me to be a good steward and honor the responsibility over all you've given me."

Mental Accountability

Reclaim yourself. Who do you want to be when you grow up? What were your goals and dreams as a young girl? Nurture yourself, ambitions, and dreams. Put as much time energy and effort into yourself as you put into others. Nurture your passions and gifts. Take time to accomplish your goals and dreams. This builds your self-confidence.

Go back to school, take that poetry class, do self-enrichment workshops. You must take time to step away from the everyday grind and give yourself a break. Go on a vacation if you can afford to. There were many times I went to the movies by myself. I've gotten hotel rooms just to take a bubble bath. Yes, I can do that at home for free. But at home there are distractions, kids, pets, chores, and so much more. A hotel room is a retreat and break from the norm and you don't have to worry about cooking or cleaning.

It's about time to fit YOU into your life. If you don't make time for yourself, how do you expect anyone else to? Don't take your mental health for granted. That's why a lot of women have nervous breakdowns or panic attacks. We go, go, go and never take time to check in on ourselves.

Emotional Accountability

Let go of all the anger, hurt, fear, guilt, and worthlessness. I had all of that bottled in me. I had to forgive. I was killing myself inside by holding on to those feelings, but trying to be *normal*. I had to define my own normal. I had to think and not let my emotions get the best of me anymore. I started taking time to love myself, this took up space so I no longer allowed the wrong man in my life. I stopped looking for love in all the wrong places.

This builds your self-esteem. You are in a higher place within yourself than you've been in the past. When you release the wrong emotions, the right feelings can manifest. It's like taking a deep breath. The longer you hold your breath, the more uncomfortable you are. Once you inhale and exhale you feel relief. You suddenly start to realize all that build-up wasn't preserving your happiness, it was preventing you from finding and enjoying it.

Soul Accountability

I had to do inventory on my life and let go of every bad habit I had picked up to survive. Like not saying "no", trying to be a people pleaser. So scared I won't have any friends, that I've accepted the wrong friends.

I had to let go of everything and everyone that was sucking the life out of me. If they are not supportive of building me up, they shouldn't be in my life.

I began looking in the mirror and saying, "You're beautiful, you're worthy, you're amazing, you're a child of God. If God be for me who can be against me?"

Whomever is against you, it doesn't matter. They have to get through God first. I serve a Mighty God, so I don't need to worry about them. I'll pray for them. Peace!

As women, we often think silence is strength, but you must release this from your being. Get a counselor or advisor, someone who can guide you positively.

Body Accountability

No more wallowing in self-pity. No more sitting around holding on to weight.

I stopped having my "Professor Klump Days"— those are days I sit around and eat any and every junk food I can find. No more ice cream, alcohol, or staying up late. No more turning to sex, that adrenaline rush for comfort. None of that is healthy and will only cause more problems.

I started exercising. Every exercise isn't for everyone. Find what gets you motivated. I like yoga, walking, elliptical, trampoline, and aerobics DVD's.

Don't give up because it didn't happen fast enough. Keep trying and stay focused on what you have accomplished. I had to fight for myself, so this diamond could emerge. Diamonds are just like women —formed under pressure, multifaceted, flawed in some areas, but absolutely priceless.

Put that nice outfit on that you've been waiting for a special occasion to wear. Fix yourself up, comb your hair, spray on your smell goods, and take yourself out on the town—dinner and a movie.

God has places He wants to send you, you can't always take a crowd. Get comfortable in the skin you're in. Yes, you're going to have nay-sayers or haters. Your family and close friends will say ugly things. People who hung out with you before will not understand or except the changes. That's absolutely alright. This is your journey.

This enforces a positive self-image. The better you think of yourself, the better you carry yourself. Do you remember when you were growing up and the elder ladies would say, "Act like a lady." This is the time to be a lady and reclaim all forms of your femininity.

Embrace all your curves but in an age appropriate non-sexual way, with confidence and pride.

Financial Accountability

Stop unnecessary spending. Stop giving your money to people who don't value you. Instead, take time to volunteer and help others. Establish steady stable cash flow. Create a budget and stick to it. Give your tithes to God and donate to causes that you're passionate about.

Save, save, save! You always want to be prepared for a rainy day or a spontaneous trip. I separated my bill account from my spending account. That way I don't go into the negative waiting for bills to clear.

This is a tangible view of the fruits of your labor. This builds a sense of independence, married or single. I'm not saying go against what works for your marriage. I'm saying be purposeful about your responsibility towards your finances.

Shalita Randall

Growing up, my mom always depended on the wolf. We were always poor, even when she worked she gave her paycheck to him. After being with him for over thirty years, she didn't have a pot to piss in or a window to throw it out of. When you feel like you are financially dependent on someone else, it can put you in desperate situations and have you at a disadvantage.

The Bible says in Proverbs 18:21, "Life and death lies in the power of thy tongue." Why are we so quick to speak death over our finances? I hear women say, "Girl I'm broke." I've heard 'I'm broke' so many times growing up, I don't like that word. We say it and then wear it like it's a badge of honor. We need to take this word out of our vocabulary when it comes to money. I don't say that word about my money.

I declare what the Bible says, God supplies all my needs through His riches and glory by Christ Jesus (Philippians 4:19). I am the head and not the tail (Deuteronomy 28:13). The Lord is my Shepherd I shall not want (Psalm 23:1).

When someone asks for money and I'm not able to give, I simply say, "No, I have money to pay my bills." Or "I'm in a financial rebuild right now, I'll see what I can do later."

Stop saying the 'b' word, it's not cute, and don't dare brag about having bad credit. We live in a world where information is a fingertip away. There are ways to rebuild credit and get budget advice.

You always want to have options, that's what money does. It opens options for you. Money also helps set a better foundation for your children to stand on. It's not about spoiling them, it's about building generational success.

The Bible says in Romans 12:2, "Be ye transformed by the renewing of your mind." Transformation does not occur without work. It takes a conscious effort to undo the habits the subconscious has adopted for your survival.

Taking control of all areas of your being helps you build your gift. It takes focus off your packaging. Taking time for you, takes power and control from all those wrongs in your life. You rebuild from the inside out, gives you power over yourself. All powerful women have found a balance in all areas of their beings.

Spiritual, mental, emotional, spiritual, physical, and financial growth after crisis is a continual work in progress. Each step of this journey is a process. Don't get stuck on the process and inhibit the progress. If you make a mistake or digress, get up, dust yourself off, and try again. Walk with confidence, smile, hold your head up, you are more than your mistakes.

I'm still on my journey, every day is an opportunity to do better than I did yesterday. No one will ever be perfect, if we were, God wouldn't have had to send Jesus.

When God created Eve in the Garden of Eden, she was whole. When He presented her to Adam she was a complete woman, from the inside out. Eve completed Adam's experience with God, woman was created to be man's helpmate. That's why the Bible says in Proverbs 18:22, "He that findeth a wife finds a good thing."

We were created to be a good thing. Not worry warts, naggers, not desperately seeking a man, not punching bags, not welcome mats or whatever society has placed on us. Throughout the Bible from the Old Testament to the New Testament, there are women mentioned and celebrated for owning their own journeys. For walking their own walks of faith and being obedient to God. God loves a praying woman vulnerable and open to the direction of the Holy Spirit.

I know my gift is so much more than my packaging. Think about this—at Christmas no matter how pretty the wrapping paper or how it's wrapped, people just tear through it. When the gift is right, they cherish it for years, a lifetime, or even generations.

As women, that's ultimately what we want—to be cherished and appreciated. I am MORE than my vagina. My gift is more valuable than my packaging.

Chapter Nine

You Are Enough: A Story of Divorce

by Diane Traenkle, DO

> *We must be willing to let go of the life we planned to have the life that is waiting for us.*
>
> *E.M. Forster*

The bright sunshine warmed my face and shoulders as I entered the church which was surrounded by a fresh blanket of sparkling white snow. The excitement of the day was intoxicating. I was about to marry the love of my life, my soul mate, the one who understands the deepest recesses of my being. The man I trusted would truly be a perfect partner and the father of my future children.

Fast forward 16 years. The naive visions of a perfect union had been replaced with the reality of deception, contempt, and heart break. In reality, I found I gave him more credit than he deserved. The man I thought I married was in fact a shell of a man full of self loathing and unresolved internal conflict.

I thought my husband adored me and respected me as an equal in our union. He bragged about my successes and virtues to our friends. He gave me accolades in public for my skill at work and my capacity as a mother and wife; whereas privately, my husband had the ability to gradually erode my self-confidence, my sense of self-worth, and my ability to believe that I could manage anything without him directing every aspect of my life. I allowed him to convince me that I was not enough.

As with many abusive relationships, I was an excellent actor in public, as was he. We attended church every Sunday, our children were very well behaved and well spoken, we were financially successful, and we showed our affection for each other. We were unstoppable.

Little did I, and everyone else know, our foundation was weak and crumbling. As my husband became more successful, he became more demanding of me. I wasn't home enough, so I scaled back my workload. Then I wasn't making enough money, so I increased my workload. I spent too much time with the kids and not enough with him, so I tried to plan date nights. He became more distant. We went to marriage seminars, he refused to follow advice, and his drinking became more noticeably excessive.

Then the bomb dropped. He had an affair with a babysitter who was half his age. All those hopes and dreams of living a full life with my soul mate crashed. That moment was the beginning of the rest of my life.

I was forced to face the daunting task of my reinvention, my recognition of inner strength, and my overcoming of fears that had been systematically inserted into my subconscious over the years.

≫⊪ ≫⊪ ≫⊪

The six months of attempting to reconcile was a story of turmoil and torture. I was fearful of letting go of my former life. It took six months to realize that my attempt to salvage the marriage was indeed one-sided. There are specific times that had significant impact on my future and my ability to survive and thrive. In retrospect, I identified three mantras or behaviors that kept me true to myself and my children. I also identified 5 major sources of fear that I needed to overcome to successfully reach the other side of the mountain, and to weather the storm in the process.

Many on the surface would think that "being replaced by a younger version" would be the worst of the situation. However, that was minor compared to the fears that lurked below while I peeled back the layers of my marriage. These fears are of the existential type. They include fear of the impact of divorce on the children, fear of shame and being judged by those around me, fear of financial instability, fear of loneliness, and the fear of retribution.

Once I came to terms with the reality of the demise of my marriage, I developed goals and mantras to get me through the lowest points.

Realization #1: Survival was the first challenge I faced during the process of realization that I was in the beginning of the fight of my life, and I could not do it alone. Fear can be crippling, and I refused to let myself be overcome by my fear. My Mantra became "be still."

Realization #2: The next revelation was to develop a 'mission statement' for myself, and subsequently my children. The goal was to teach my kids to value a life that brings peace and contentment.

Realization #3: Lastly, I needed a mantra to remind me of the importance of accountability and remaining true to myself and my family. My mantra was to remind myself that instant gratification feels good now, but delayed gratification feels good for a lifetime.

⯈⯈ ⯈⯈ ⯈⯈

Before I filed for divorce, I visited my friend, Aya (the compiler of this wonderful anthology you are reading). I went to see Aya for the dedication of her fifth child. She was unaware of the circumstances of my marital problems until I told her my husband was not coming with me. At the time, he was convinced by his office manager to check himself into an inpatient rehab for alcohol abuse. Friends convinced me to visit Aya anyway so that I was not tempted to get him out. That was also the same week that the secret of the affair went public.

I spent a long weekend with Aya's family, crying most of the time because I was getting threatening texts and phone calls from my husband the entire time. Aya was a life saver in that she was able to organize the events of the weekend and take care of her friend who was falling apart at the seams. When she dropped me off at the airport to return home, Aya gave me Joyce Meyer's book, "Peace: Cast All Your Cares Upon Him."

My husband had left the rehab center three days after arriving and was on his way back home, against the advice of the counselors at the center. As I was traveling home, he told me not to come home because I didn't belong there anymore.

I read that book two times on the way home and underlined parts that resonated with me. Aya was my angel that day. I don't think I would have had the courage to go back home if she hadn't given me that book. I repeatedly read the page that described how Jesus could help us weather any storm as long as we focus on Him. I was in the middle of my own storm. I used the passage as a meditation focus point and kept myself calm.

I went back home, where I belonged. In finding a focal point and recognizing that I was carrying an incredibly heavy burden, I was able to rise up to a level of existence that made me strong enough to have the courage to move forward during the divorce process, no matter how much I was threatened.

As it became more apparent that my marriage would fail, I decided to consult with an attorney about divorce. In our first meeting, I let him know that my goals at the end of this ordeal were to maintain my integrity and help my children survive the divorce as well as I can. I told him I needed him to remember my goals so that he could remind me if I begin to stray from my path. I made sure I had a group of friends surrounding me who all knew my goals so that they could hold me accountable and help me maintain my path as well.

The week before I filed for divorce, my husband presented me with papers from a lawyer he hired to get a 'speedy' divorce, which included a joint custody agreement. I didn't read the papers. I just stared at them, speechless. He was really pushing the joint custody line. I pretended to not be familiar with the set up and stalled by telling him I would like to get a lawyer and discuss options since he seemed to know more than I did. He agreed, but continued to harass me for the next few days. It was the week between Christmas and New Year, so the court house and law offices were closed.

One night my husband was particularly impatient. It happened to be New Year's Eve. We pretended to be happy for the kids until they went to bed. He then cornered me in our bedroom (he was sleeping in a spare room by then) and proceeded to pressure me into signing the papers. I think he was becoming suspicious that I knew what I was doing because he then said something that haunts me to this day: "If you file for divorce and file for full custody, I promise I will take away your kids, your house, and your job."

The look of contempt on his face was terrifying. How could someone I loved and I thought loved me be so hateful and threatening? The effects of fear took over my body and my mind. My heart was racing and pounding out of my chest. I had a knot in my throat. My feet and hands grew cold. My body shook. My breath was taken away. My mind raced as I considered how bleak my future may become. I was stunned to silence. I did not sleep that night; the first of many hyper-vigilant sleepless nights.

However, I was convicted to file first and file for full custody, knowing full well that he will try his hardest to fulfill his promise, and he sure did try. The storm that raged around me gave me the resolve to focus on the stillness of Jesus as He carried me through the hurricane. I was not doing this alone.

How do we overcome the crippling fear that is caused by abusers' threats combined with our own personal insecurities? That Joyce Meyer book sure did get a lot of wear and tear through that time of my life.

I prayed, I relied on close friends, my pastor, and I cried a whole lot in the shower. What worked very well was always having a plan of action. Always doing something to improve my situation, whether it be counseling, exercise, talking with close friends, walking, or planning strategy with my attorney.

I had to remain focused, even though my husband was about to launch an attack on everything dear to me. My fear of what he was capable of caused me to make decisions that may not have been the best at the time. After all, I was really in a fight for my life and the lives of my children. Let me explain those fears.

The Kids

"The most profound thing we have to offer our children is our own healing." - Anne Lamott

I used my kids as an excuse to explain why I wasn't leaving the marriage. Many women verbalize the reason they stay with an abusive spouse is because they need to keep the family together for the kids. What makes us fear breaking up a family? Are we really breaking up a family, or are we helping the family heal? Are we blaming ourselves for the behavior of our spouse? It sure sounds like it, in retrospect.

I was afraid of parenting alone, despite the fact that I was already parenting with little help. I was afraid the kids would hate me for getting a divorce because they may never know the true reason why I had to do what I did. Will the kids become emotionally unstable because of my choice to divorce their father? What will their father tell them about me?

First I had to accept that I was not keeping the family together for the kids. I was doing it because I was afraid. The day I realized the truth was the day my then 13-year-old daughter, who was unaware of her dad's infidelity, got angry at me and asked me why her father was still around.

"Why is he here? He is mean to you, he doesn't take care of you, he doesn't take care of us. Why don't you just kick him out?" She said.

After I filed for divorce and my husband moved out, things got a bit dangerous—stalking, chasing me around the house in front of the kids, lunging at me, threatening me, etc. Even with all of that, I yet still felt a weight lifted off my shoulders after filing for divorce. I knew I made the right choice, not only for myself, but for my kids.

I realized I was very good at parenting, especially without the extra burden of resentment when I was not helped. Since my role as a wife was gone, I was able to elevate my role as a mom. I put them directly into counseling after we told all the kids about the divorce, knowing that their father was going to lie to them about many things. I made sure we followed routines to try to control the chaos, which is especially important if living arrangements change. I spent time with each of the kids at bed time to pray with them, tell them how important they are to me and how smart they are. We talked about our day and I answered questions to the best of my ability. I was scripted by their counselor to answer the tough questions.

I actually was very proud of how I was able to step up. To this day I truly believe that I am a better, more intentional parent than if I was still married.

Children need structure, unconditional love, respect, peace, and trust in their lives. They are resilient. I don't know how many times I heard the word resilient, but it was so true. We have new traditions that they hold sacred. My kids feel safe when they are with me. So safe that I get the wrath of my son's temper now and again because he knows I provide unconditional love.

In leaving a bad marriage, I was able to model independence, courage, self respect, and maintaining boundaries. I had goals, and I had focus. I also learned to forgive myself when I screwed up because there were plenty of mistakes and no one is perfect.

I made myself a mantra that kept me in line when I became upset at the snail's pace of my recovery and the return to some sort of normalcy in my life and the lives of my children. In the past, I observed other people impulsively acting out to try to help themselves escape or feel better. I realized that impulsivity left people, including my ex-husband, empty inside. I wanted to remain a good role model for my children, therefore I repeated this to myself many times: instant gratification feels good now, but delayed gratification feels good for a lifetime.

Finances

Next on the fear list was finances. Can I afford to go it alone? Do I have job security? Will I be able to do my job safely and effectively with all this stress? How will I pay for the legal fees? What possessions will I lose?

Getting divorced is similar to a house fire in that you risk losing everything. There is so much uncertainty, but after a while, there is a realization that money can't buy that which is truly valuable— health, kids, love. But you still need to live so you still need a source of income. My delayed gratification mantra kept me in line many a times when I was trying to figure out finances.

Many women who are in abusive situations have an issue with boundaries. One of the common mistakes I heard was women gave up and let the spouse walk all over them during a divorce process. However, this is the time to stick up for yourself—be proactive and anticipatory, make a budget, learn to keep to it and get reliable financial advice. If friends or family offer help, take them up on it.

Women often give up careers to raise their kids, not anticipating ever having to support themselves in the future. There is power with going back and creating a career, whether it entails doing something completely new, or going back to school.

Trying to keep it together at work is so hard when your personal life is falling apart. I had to force myself to compartmentalize, forgive myself, and pace myself. I was blessed with support and understanding from my colleagues and my administrators.

Loneliness

One of my self-care activities was bike riding. On a warm afternoon I found myself riding on a path in a wooded park in town. I passed a family of four who had stopped for a rest. They were obviously enjoying the day and each other's company. That scene destroyed me a little inside. I wept uncontrollably the rest of the bike ride. I was angry and sad. Not just for myself, but for my kids as well. We had that happy scene stolen from us. I will never get to experience a peaceful afternoon with my children and their father again.

We were social beings. We thrived on companionship. The loss of that companionship was devastating, even if the marriage was not healthy. Who do I talk to about what happened at work? Who will hug me when I am down? Will I ever have intimacy again?

So let's reframe loneliness and turn it into solitude. That took a very long time to do. I had to learn to be able to love myself enough to build myself up and arm myself against loneliness. I worked hard to arm myself with the belief that I am enough. My mantra on delayed gratification helped me a great deal to remember that my decisions will impact my future as well as the future and welfare of my children.

I used to cry every time I dropped the kids off to their father's apartment in the beginning of the divorce process. I was not confident in his parenting skills and he was verbally abusive towards my oldest. Plus I knew I was going home to an empty, quiet house. For the first few months, I would drive to a friend's house and cry for a few hours, then go home after my friend built me back up again.

Eventually I learned how to keep myself from breaking down. I made a bucket list of everything I wanted to do. After seeing how much was on my list, I decided I'd better get started. I learned that hobbies (mine was photography) not only help the time pass, but a hobby also builds up self-esteem that had eroded away from the years of allowing myself to be convinced I had no value.

I found that finding a passion was putting a smile on my face. I found peace in the storm. I learned the difference between loneliness and solitude. After being by myself, I became fond of the solitude. I was able to become self-aware, redefine myself, learn the importance of loving myself. After coming to grips with the reality that I could not control what happened on his visitation time with the kids, my perspective changed from losing my kids for a weekend to having a "free" sitter so that I can do things that I was never able to do because I never had a break like this before.

The surprising outcome from this solitude was that I got so comfortable being by myself that I found myself having to adjust to the kids being back when they were gone for more than a few days. They had to adjust as well.

I learned the value of having trusted friends/family member(s) to commune. Good relationships promote good health. A memory in particular had to do with the fact that one of my dearest friends to this day will still tell me she loves me. I am forever in awe of her awareness of the fact that I would need to hear someone besides my kids say those simple words to me.

Shame

Despite the fact that divorce is so prevalent, there is still a stigma attached to it—you are damaged goods. I failed at marriage, I carried blame. I felt my character was being judged. I was my worst critic. Marriage is supposed to be forever. I was a great pretender in my marriage. From the outside, we looked like a perfect family. Watching the shock and disappointment from others was painful.

The burden of shame is too heavy for one person to bear. I found myself relying on God to help me shoulder the burden. I also realized that I had nothing to be ashamed of. I had to recognize my integrity and my strength in order to recognize that what eventually broke the marriage was not my burden to carry. I don't have to fake it anymore.

Opening up to those close to me and admitting my weakness to God helped relieve enough of the burden that I felt it physically lift from me. As the burden lifted, I was able to think more clearly, and able to see brightness in my future. This made it more possible to take better care of myself, and therefore my children as well as my career.

Retaliation

Retaliation can be emotional, financial, and physical. This can be a real, life-threatening fear. The week I filed for divorce, I also took my husband off my life insurance, my will, and got all of my finances organized. Again, I was afraid of what my ex-husband was capable of. There were times in the first few months when I was forced to call the police, call women's aid service for advice, and go into hiding. I became hyper-vigilant.

I lost about 40 pounds (don't worry, I found it again). My heart rate was mostly above 100 and I had a visceral reaction to anything that resembled the sound of the garage door opening. I was fully aware of the fact that there are two times when an abused woman is most likely to be killed: during pregnancy and when she is trying to leave the relationship.

Fortunately for me, I was not a victim of physical violence, most likely because he was focused on his relationship with our former babysitter. It took months for me not to panic when I heard the sound of a garage door open. It took years for me not to have a panic response to seeing him. I focused on maintaining my peace by meditation and prayer. I also made sure that there was never a situation where I would be alone with him and I avoided confrontations.

Any communication was regarding child issues. If he tried to engage me in a confrontation, I would shut the conversation down and show him distinct boundaries that I was never brave enough to show before. As my self-confidence grew, my fear began to dissipate because I realized that losing my fear empowered me.

As the dissolution of my marriage began to unfold, I set goals and shared them with others. I wanted to maintain my integrity, and I wanted my kids to get through our nightmare intact. I also wanted to reach a point of peace and contentment that I lacked in my life.

I was gifted with books by friends, most notably Joyce Meyer's book "Peace: Cast All Your Cares Upon Him", which became my constant companion when I felt I was becoming overwhelmed with grief, fear, and helplessness. I was reminded of the fact that I am not facing this adversity alone. The mantra of staying true to myself kept me on my path of integrity. It is so easy to stray when there are so many temptations, but the easy path is rarely the right path.

Fear is overcome by action, faith, self-care, letting go of anger, separation from the cause of the fear, and gaining confidence. I was forced to reinvent myself, but in the end, I realized that all I did was get "me" back. I realized that fear restricted my progress to my goals. There is no quick or easy way to heal. There is no formula or one-size-fits-all way to thrive after divorce. But there is always our God who is more than willing to share our burden and help us through the inevitable storms of life.

I've been overwhelmed, beaten down, I've cried many times in the shower. I've beaten up the inside of my car wailing from the grief. But then I get myself together and keep moving forward.

I am reminded of a passage from Mitch Albom's book, Tuesdays with Morrie: An Old Man, a Young Man, and Life's Greatest Lesson.[11] When Morrie is asked how he makes a choice to be positive every single day even though he is dying, he explains that he allows himself a few minutes to feel sorry for himself, then he picks himself up and resolves to be happy.

Sometimes it takes a monumental crisis to make you realize that you are enough.

 THE END

Meet the Authors

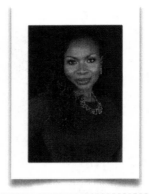

Aya Fubara Eneli, Esq.
Pioneer Author of Live Your Abundant Life Too

Aya Fubara Eneli is an attorney, best-selling author, certified life coach, and inspirational speaker, with clients in thirteen countries. She is an alumnus of The Ohio State University, where she gained her Juris Doctorate and a Master's in African/African American Studies, as well as two other degrees, and is featured in An Encyclopedia of Path-breaking Women at The Ohio State University.

Aya is passionate about family, her faith and social justice. Her life's purpose statement is to empower and equip individuals to live to their highest potential. She has been married to her husband, Dr. Kenechukwu Eneli, since 1997, and together they have five children, three of whom are entrepreneurs. To learn more, visit her website at **www.ayaeneli.com**

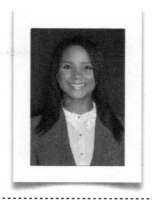

Keiko Anderson, Esq.

Keiko Anderson, Esquire is the proud mother of Camille Griffin (16), Jasmine Anderson (21), and Calvin Anderson (22). She is the proud wife of Reverend Dr. Colonel DeVry Anderson. She was born and raised in San Antonio, Texas, but has lived most of her adult life in Austin.

Keiko obtained a Bachelors in Social Work in 1999 from the University of Texas at Austin; and a Doctors of Jurisprudence from the University of Texas Law School in 2003. In 2005, Keiko began her law practice, the Law Office of Keiko Griffin, as a solo practitioner; and has been in operation for over 13 years.

In her time away from home and work, Keiko devotes her time ministering to women and children through church organizations and conferences.

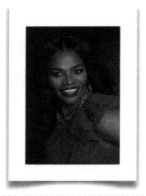

Nicola Myers Gardere

An accomplished administrator, teacher, mother and scholar, Nicola Myers Gardere is an Assistant Principal at Manor Middle School in Killeen, Texas. She has presented at the National Conference of Black School Educators with a focus on Poetry in Motion and 21st Century Learners. She has also served as the guest speaker at various charitable organizations in the community to bring awareness to the importance of educating our youths. Nicola is a servant leader in her community and volunteers with countless organizations.

Nicola has earned a Bachelor of Science in Human Services Management as well as a Masters in Curriculum and Instruction. She is currently pursuing a course of study leading to a Doctor of Education in Administration Leadership.

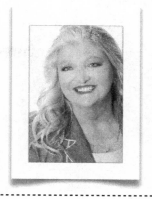

Laura L. Johnson

Laura L. Johnson is an Army military police veteran; Founder/CEO of Malakai Heavens Missions; Leadership Trainer Celebrate Recovery; blogger of "Better Not Bitter"; church seeder in Nairobi; overcomer of domestic violence, early childhood sodomy, teen rape, military rape, abortion and suicide.

A believer and follower of Jesus Christ, Laura is strong-willed, soft-hearted and loyal. Believing "through God ALL things are possible", Laura stands for moral, civil and social justice for all regardless of gender, race, color or religion.

Teaching and counseling in Celebrate Recovery for many years, Laura believes only God can repair the broken and disconnected pieces of our soul.

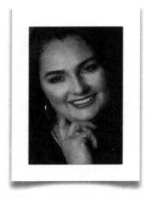

Brigette Marie

Born in south-side Chicago, Illinois, Brigette Marie overcame being raised in an environment of abuse, alcoholism, drug addiction and poverty. She is a proud single mother of three amazing young men; and the only child of her biological parents to become a college graduate. Brigette also served almost 11 years in the United States Army, with deployments to Bosnia and Iraq.

Brigette is currently pursuing her Masters of Science in Nursing in Health Care Management and Business Administration. When her children have graduated high school and moved forward independently pursuing their dreams, Brigette plans to be a part of world-wide medical missions with an organization called "Nurses Without Borders".

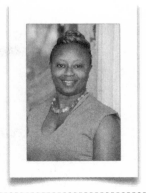

Shalita Randall

Shalita Randall is a God-fearing woman and mother of one son. She is the only veteran and college graduate in her family, which she is one of ten children. Born and raised in Houston, Texas, Shalita grew up in a poverty-stricken home. She joined the Army in 2001 which afforded her the opportunity to go to for school for respiratory therapy. Shalita worked at Darnall Army Medical Center on the Ft. Hood Army base, from 2009 until medical retirement in 2018.

Shalita's dream of being a published author came true when she met the incredible Aya Eneli, who has been a friend, a guide, a coach, and an inspiration to her life. Through Aya, Shalita is an active participant in Aya's foundation—the Intelligent and Talented Girls, where they mentor and lead young girls ages 11-17.

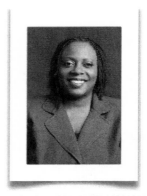

Vannette P. Simmons

Vannette P. Simmons is a first-generation American, a United States Army veteran, and a Gold Star wife who was born in Brooklyn, New York. She has two children, Ahmari and Elon, who owns her own tutoring company.

Vannette has been a passionate educator for the past 10 years. She earned her Bachelor of Science in Computer Science from Claflin University in South Carolina; and a Master of Science in Education with a specialization in Integrating Technology in the Classroom from Walden University.

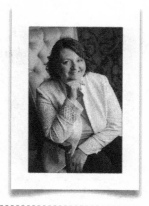

Diane Traenkle, DO

Diane Traenkle is a practicing physician specializing in Obstetrics and Gynecology in mid-Michigan. She is also an adjunct professor at Central Michigan University in the Physician Assistant Program.

Diane is the proud mother of five children (age range from adolescent to adult). She received a Bachelor of Science in Biology from the University of Scranton, and Doctor of Osteopathy from the University of New England College of Osteopathic Medicine. Her residency training was through Michigan State University.

Diane is a lover of nature, an avid explorer, and is never without her camera.

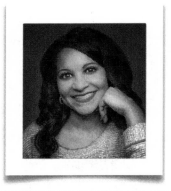

Amber N. Warner

Amber N. Warner is a Licensed Clinical Social Worker, with over 20 years of experience. She studied under the direction of Dr. David Burns, leading Psychiatrist and adjunct professor at Stanford University, and the developer of TEAM—a new form of Cognitive Behavioral Therapy for the treatment of depression and anxiety. She has achieved Level 2 TEAM certification from the Feeling Good Institute. Amber also has a certification from the National Clearinghouse on Families and Youth in Trauma-Informed Care.

Most of all, Amber has a passion for people, their wellness, and quality of life. She currently resides in California; enjoys spending time with family and friends, hiking, Inferno Pilates, learning new things, traveling, community service, attending church, and an occasional new pair of shoes.

Footnotes

[1] Shepherd, S. R. (2014). *His princess: Love letters from your king*. Colorado Springs, CO: Multnomah Books.

[2] Martin, C. (1994). *Creating a positive self-image: Celebrating the uniqueness of you*. DVD published by Christine Martin Ministries.

[3] Craft, K. (2014, October 7). *Your divine fingerprint: The force that makes you unstoppable*. New York, NY: HarperOne.

[4] Cloud, H. & Townsend, J. (2000, February 21). *Boundaries in dating: How healthy choices grow healthy relationships*. Grand Rapids, MI: Zondervan.

[5] Hirsch, E. (2016, March 1). *Gabriel: A poem*. New York, NY: Knopf, Division of Random House LLC.

[6] Covey, S.R. (2013, November 19). *The 7 habits of highly effective people: Powerful lessons in personal change*. New York, NY: Simon & Schuster.

[7] . Fogel, A. (2012, April 19). Emotional and Physical Pain Activate Similar Brain Regions: Where Does Emotion Hurt in the Body? *Psychology Today*. Retrieved from https://www.psychologytoday.com/us/blog/body-sense/201204/emotional-and-physical-pain-activate-similar-brain-regions

8. Wolfelt, Alan D., Ph.D. (2016, December 14). The Journey Through Grief: The Six Needs of Mourning. *Center for Loss and Transition*. Retrieved at https://www.centerforloss.com/2016/12/journey-grief-six-needs-mourning/

9. Tousley, Marty, RN, MS, FT, BC-TMH. (2018, March 27). Finding Crying Time in Grief. Retrieved at https://www.griefhealingblog.com/2013/12/finding-crying-time-in-grief.html

10. Mayo Foundation for Medical Education and Research. (2018). Broken Heart Syndrome. Retrieved at https://www.mayoclinic.org/diseases-conditions/broken-heart-syndrome/symptoms-causes/syc-20354617

11 Albom, M. (2002, October 8). *Tuesdays with Morrie: An old man, a young man, and life's greatest lesson, 20th anniversary edition*. New York, NY: Broadway Books.

18996552R00136

Made in the USA
San Bernardino, CA
21 December 2018